T0276755

# Spiritual Fertility

## Hay House Titles of Related Interest

*YOU CAN HEAL YOUR LIFE, the movie,*
starring Louise Hay & Friends
(available as a 1-DVD program, an expanded
2-DVD set, and an online streaming video)
Watch the trailer at: www.hayhouse.com/louise-movie

*THE SHIFT, the movie,*
starring Dr. Wayne W. Dyer
(available as a 1-DVD program, an expanded
2-DVD set, and on online streaming video)
Watch the trailer at: www.hayhouse.com/the-shift-movie

*EVERYTHING IS HERE TO HELP YOU: Finding the
Gift in Life's Greatest Challenges,* by Matt Kahn

*LIFE ON EARTH: Understanding Who We Are, How We
Got Here, and What May Lie Ahead,* by Mike Dooley

*LIGHT IS THE NEW BLACK: A Guide to Answering Your Soul's
Callings and Working Your Light,* by Rebecca Campbell

*MAKING LIFE EASY: How the Divine Inside Can Heal Your
Body and Your Life,* by Christiane Northrup, M.D.

*RAISE YOUR VIBRATION: 111 Practices to Increase
Your Spiritual Connection,* by Kyle Gray

*THE UNIVERSE HAS YOUR BACK: Transform
Fear to Faith,* by Gabrielle Bernstein

All of the above are available at your local bookstore
or may be ordered by visiting:

Hay House USA: www.hayhouse.com®
Hay House Australia: www.hayhouse.com.au
Hay House UK: www.hayhouse.co.uk
Hay House India: www.hayhouse.co.in

# Spiritual Fertility

DR. JULIE VON

*Integrative Practices for the Journey to Motherhood*

**HAY HOUSE, INC.**
Carlsbad, California • New York City
London • Sydney • New Delhi

Copyright © 2019 by Dr. Julie Von

*Published in the United States by:* Hay House, Inc.: www.hayhouse
.com® • *Published in Australia by:* Hay House Australia Pty. Ltd.: www
.hayhouse.com.au • *Published in the United Kingdom by:* Hay House
UK, Ltd.: www.hayhouse.co.uk • *Published in India by:* Hay House Publishers India: www.hayhouse.co.in

*Cover design:* Jordan Wannemacher    •    *Interior design:* Joe Bernier

All rights reserved. No part of this book may be reproduced by any
mechanical, photographic, or electronic process, or in the form of a pho-
nographic recording; nor may it be stored in a retrieval system, trans-
mitted, or otherwise be copied for public or private use—other than for
"fair use" as brief quotations embodied in articles and reviews—without
prior written permission of the publisher.

The author of this book does not dispense medical advice or pre-
scribe the use of any technique as a form of treatment for physical, emotional, or medical problems without the advice of a physician, either
directly or indirectly. The intent of the author is only to offer information of a general nature to help you in your quest for emotional,
physical, and spiritual well-being. In the event you use any of the information in this book for yourself, the author and the publisher assume
no responsibility for your actions.

All names and identifying details of have been changed to protect
their privacy.

Lyrics to "Calling In (Fill Up My Mojo)" by Donna Lewis have been
used with permission.

**Cataloging-in-Publication Data is on file at the Library of Congress**

**Tradepaper ISBN:** 978-1-4019-5623-3
**e-book ISBN:** 978-1-4019-5624-0

10  9  8  7  6  5  4  3  2  1
1st edition, July 2019

Printed in the United States of America

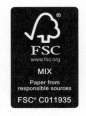
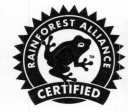

*For Scott and Anna Libertine*

# Contents

*Introduction: The Heart of the Matter*............................................ix

## Chapter 1
The New Conception: Energy before Matter .............................. 1

## Chapter 2
Transgenerational Trauma and the
Trauma Surrounding Our Births ............................................. 23

## Chapter 3
Psychological and Energetic
Blocks to Becoming Pregnant.................................................. 49

## Chapter 4
The Impact of Our Most Intimate
Relationships on Our Fertility.................................................. 69

## Chapter 5
Transforming Limiting Beliefs ................................................. 87

## Chapter 6
The Unconscious as Healer...................................................... 107

## Chapter 7
Symbols, Synchronicity, and Cosmic Timing........................... 125

## Chapter 8
How Our Ancestors and Spirit Guides
Aid in the Fertility Journey ..................................................... 143

## Chapter 9
Karmic Connections, Spirit Contracts, and Past Lives ........... 165

## Chapter 10
The Power of Prayer ................................................................. 185

*Conclusion: The Future of Fertility* .............................................. 203
*Acknowledgments* ......................................................................... 213
*About the Author* .......................................................................... 217

# Introduction

# The Heart of the Matter

This book started with the inspiration to help more people. After years of clinical practice, and after witnessing patient after patient compliantly doing everything right both in Western medicine and holistic medicine and yet still not being able to have children, I radically changed the way I practiced medicine. I flipped my own narrative and returned to my roots of energetic and spiritual healing.

The issue at the heart of the fertility problem became clear to me. The freedom that has come from individualization, sexual liberation, and moral and religious freedom has provided us with multiple paths of choice for self-actualization. At the same time, modernity has overstimulated our nervous systems, and our endocrine systems have gone haywire in response. What we have inadvertently developed is a culture of hypervigilance.

I began to ask how I could teach an individual to let go, trust, and relax into the process of conceiving. How could I give even the most cynical of my patients a system of spiritual beliefs that allowed them to release their vigilance and balance their endocrine system? How could I empower people to return to their intuitive wisdom as a powerful tool for healing fertility?

The vision of *Spiritual Fertility* hit me two years before I wrote this book. I was still navigating my own questions about how my colleagues and friends, especially the ones in the medical community, would perceive me if I wrote about my method and practice of integrating intuition, faith, and spiritual science. I had worked very hard as an integrative doctor to be seen as an equal with the predominant allopathic medicine community. I tried to avoid writing this book, but something felt destined about it—and I could no longer sit back and not share my highly effective clinical observations.

In this time, what I call my reconstructive period after I had lived through the dismantling of my identity that comes with motherhood, I returned full circle to my own spiritual practices. I said a prayer to Saint Michael, asking to help and support me in finding a path for my message to be delivered to the world. And I swore an oath to write this book, no matter how long or difficult the path.

To my surprise, soon after this oath, a sequence of events occurred that led to a meeting with Hay House and a contract to write the book you hold in your hands today. Every step of the way, I was guided by spirit and intuition. What I had made impossible and difficult in my rational mind was no match for the power of the heart. Every person involved in getting this book to you, in this moment, is a testament to how powerful intuitive wisdom is and how it is ultimately an extension of a universal plan. In Chapter 8, when I speak about ancestral and spirit guides,

I mention that the ancestor who passes away close to the event of conception often becomes one of your guides. Louise Hay, one of the great crusaders of intuitive healing in modern times, passed away just before the conception of this book—and I have felt her palpable presence and support during the writing of *Spiritual Fertility*.

The intuitive and energetic support that I received in the conception and creation of this book is an extension of an entire spiritual support system that wants to be of assistance to you in your life. I think of this energy as the universe's response to the current state of fertility on the planet. According to statistics, although 60 percent of couples will conceive without medical intervention within six months of trying, one in eight couples struggles with infertility. This imbalance has not gone unseen by the Divine and although fertility is certainly in a fragile state, it too is evolving and developing in accord with a universal plan.

Infertility is defined as the inability to get pregnant or maintain a pregnancy after adequately trying for 12 months without medical intervention—and that period of time shifts depending on a woman's age. Today, 7.4 women between 15 and 44 have difficulty getting and staying pregnant; this comprises 12 percent of all women, according to reports from the U.S. Centers for Disease Control and Prevention (CDC).

Despite the rising number of women and couples turning to in vitro fertilization (IVF) and other medically invasive procedures, there are still so many unknowns when it comes to solving the so-called epidemic of infertility. Often, even when everything "looks good on paper," unseen factors intervene.

Given the sheer number of variables modern women are facing—from environmental stressors to overstimulation, to illness, to trauma, to a slew of other variables that are seldom accounted for by medical professionals— conventional medicine's tendency to paint over individual circumstances with the broad brush of infertility is not only disheartening . . . it's also inaccurate.

Everyone is fertile; however, our common standards for measuring fertility are faulty.

A woman's body is a beautiful, intricate system that is always attempting to achieve regulation. There is a vast range of tools that can help this process and correct the stressors in her life. Accessing them requires differentiating women's individual stressors and allowing them to customize solutions that will work for them.

The dynamic spark that is responsible for creating each new human being cannot be reduced to a mass of cells and biochemical processes. There is a deeper mystery at play that women who are struggling with fertility can tap into, in order to become their own empowered advocates.

## CHOOSING CONSCIENCE CONCEPTION

I wrote *Spiritual Fertility* to help women and couples dive more deeply into that mystery. This book is not about "infertility." It is about how to navigate fertility so that you don't lose your agency, making the entire experience of becoming pregnant energetically uplifting. *Spiritual Fertility* was developed as a clarion call to women who have felt discouraged or alone in their fertility journeys. It is meant to help you cultivate the sovereignty to navigate this journey and to develop a deeper relationship with a universe of untapped energies that can be accessed to your benefit.

As a holistic fertility doctor with decades of clinical experience, I have developed a groundbreaking framework for introducing tools that nourish and build women's receptive energy so that we can connect to the spiritual and unseen aspects of creating life. In my own work, I have witnessed firsthand that this spiritual path within fertility balances the hormonal system and promotes a healthy pregnancy.

This framework is the solution to our current accepted narratives around fertility, which offer much in the way of diagnoses but little in the way of customized solutions and full consideration of a woman's entire ecosystem of self: mind, body, and spirit. Children, no matter by what means they are conceived and born, carry the energetic operating system for all of us who share the future of the planet. This book reminds us, as a society, of that. In using the tools of ancient and modern spiritual and intuitive wisdom and wedding them with rational science, we can choose conscious conception over a mechanical approach. Instead of defining ourselves on the basis of our symptoms, we can use them to identify the deepest root of who we are and what we must overcome in order to bring forth new life.

*Spiritual Fertility* is a deeply compassionate guide for self-care in which the journey toward your healing also becomes the journey toward fertility. In helping you shift your emotive states and reorient with your wholeness, I want to offer you the kind of transformation that is necessary to connect with the spirits of your future children.

In this book, I infuse my own experiences as a fertility doctor and intuitive with the stories of my clients. I make the leap from the body's energetics to how we can harness our energetic connection to the universe in a practical and magical way to work with a force that hasn't occurred yet: pregnancy. You will learn how the principles of cosmic timing can be applied to all processes having to do with fertility and child-rearing—from freezing eggs, to conceiving, to choosing to adopt.

When I work with clients, we look deeply into the unconscious energies that influence their connection to reproduction, including the social, medical, and familial narratives that are sometimes blindly disseminated. I take into account fertility lab reports, as well as blood tests and menstrual cycle tracking, in addition to the subtler findings that I have been trained to observe. Sound, sight, smell, and feel all deliver valuable data as to why fertility might be stagnant, congested, or blocked. A client's choice of words, her pitch and vocalization, as well as body language and respiration all describe the history of that person's life.

I also look for the signs and synchronicities of the universe as I work with individuals. I might think back to a moment of my own life, or a past patient I worked with as I start to work with someone new. The resonance between the two provides me with insight into a pattern that they might have in common. Signs from nature—like hail, lightning, or chaotic storms—can also provide intuitive information about the energetics that might be surrounding an individual patient. Sightings of animals—such as hawks, doves, or owls—while I am speaking to a patient can prove to be powerful, revelatory data.

## CONNECTING WITH YOUR INTUITIVE WISDOM

Finding positive, supportive ways to reframe fear and stress is essential to getting pregnant. There is no one individual cause of infertility, and no individual is the cause of his or her fertility challenges. In examining the impact of such belief systems, my clients often discover the psychological and energetic blocks within their body, mind, and spirit. Many of my clients, despite the "odds," do end up conceiving by using the principles of spiritual fertility and foregoing medical "knowledge" to connect with their own intuitive wisdom.

In the current climate of the world, the keys to the sacred are not so obvious. They are hidden in the realm of the invisible, which is often forgotten and relegated to irrelevance or superstition. Unlocking these messages so that they can empower us requires developing a meditative and receptive space so we can have the silence to hear and decipher them.

*Spiritual Fertility* will be your guide for honing your intuitive skills. I am here to show every woman who undergoes challenges in her fertility journey that she is a warrior, and that she can use her strength to access integral information about her pregnancy that is just as important as her estrogen levels and her iron intake.

This book also explains how my path to developing this practice involved my own return to a more spirit-based approach to medicine. Chapter 1 offers a number of case studies of clients who have harnessed the main principles of spiritual fertility—namely, connecting to intuition and the capacity to tap into unseen forces—to empower themselves in their fertility journeys. Chapter 2 introduces the concept of trauma inherited from our ancestors, as well as trauma from our own perinatal and birth experiences, and how I have empowered my clients to overwrite harmful transgenerational narratives. Chapter 3 explores how the emotions of fear, anxiety, sadness, and worry can injure the connection between the heart and the uterus (something I call "womb break"). I also walk you through powerful exercises to heal the injuries and blockages that can be caused by miscarriage, abortion, and trauma from medical procedures. Chapter 4 explores how to connect to intuition and to energetic blockages within intimate relationships, as well as your relationship to your family and the universe. It brings to light the important role identity plays within motherhood and fertility, and how to prioritize self-care as a powerful healing act.

Chapter 5 switches from discussing more "real" and material traumas to exploring how we can work with our spirit to heal ourselves. Through intentional practices in mindfulness, it builds on the self-care you learned in the previous chapter to enable you to connect with your authentic intuitive impulses rather than learned beliefs. Chapter 6 highlights Jungian symbolism and dream interpretation as tools to identify cultural beliefs about fertility. This chapter also expands on previously covered material by discussing how dreams can deliver clear messages about unresolved blockages in fertility, as well as connecting you directly to the spirit of your unborn children. Chapter 7 teaches you how to look for signs from the transpersonal realm—which can be found in nature, and even in our immediate environments—and to connect with larger cycles of time, as described by Eastern medicine and other spiritual systems, in understanding your own fertility journey. At this point in *Spiritual Fertility*, you will have developed a good sense of your intuition and how to care for and protect it. Next we will put your intuitive insights to work as we dive into the specifics of how to connect with your spirit babies.

Chapter 8 helps you find your "upstairs team" and describes the clear steps of communicating and listening to the wisdom of benevolent energies, such as your ancestral guides. Chapter 9 delves into the more esoteric matter of karmic connections and contracts that we make before incarnating into the world—and how we can identify these contracts and communicate directly with spirit babies. Chapter 10 explores traditions around the world that effectively use prayer to help with fertility. I detail prayer's efficacy in helping women to bypass the rational mind, relax the nervous system, and align us with an incomprehensible force that can help us reach our desired objectives without strain. We conclude with some thoughts on the future of fertility, and how the adoption of the methods in this book can lead to a healthier connection with our minds, bodies, and spirits—not to mention the minds, bodies, and spirits of our children.

Within each chapter, you will find healing rituals and tools for incorporating this practical magic into your busy life. Each has been clinically tested and proven to be helpful in your fertility journey. I encourage you to complete all of the exercises in the book. Many of my clients enjoy keeping a journal of their findings and thoughts as they work through the material.

## EMBRACING ENERGETIC AND SPIRITUAL HEALING

*Spiritual Fertility* is the culmination of my many years of working with and advocating for women's reproductive health. What I have discovered, and what remains so misunderstood by conventional medicine and its proponents, is that the reasons behind women's inability to get pregnant are almost always on the level of energy rather than matter. When women learn to pay attention to the underlying dynamics behind their challenges, what they experience is nothing less than an entire shift in the field of their mind/body/spirit.

Early in my life, I received a vital glimpse of my purpose as a clinical practitioner, a spiritual advocate, and a steward of the universe's unseen forces. I believe that the practice of spiritual fertility will offer you the same magical experience of connecting with the life that has not yet taken form inside you. It is my hope that the book will offer you the tools to understand that you have the power to change your narrative about your fertility, and your life.

I am positive that spiritual fertility will help countless people envision a future that is beautiful, peaceful, healthy, and free from so many of the stressors and traumas that dictate our realities. I trust that this is a vision that will change the world.

# Chapter 1

# The New Conception: Energy before Matter

It comes like a whisper. A gold thread braided through the density and events of our lives. Yet once the thread finds you, it is undeniable: you have experienced the first imprint of a child's soul.

I became aware of my ability to sense the golden threads of attached souls somewhere around age 17, when I was given awareness of my future daughter's appearance within my field. By "attached souls," I mean that, because energy precedes matter, the timeless connections between spirits can be felt and observed in the subtle and unseen energetic fields, or auras, of each person, even before pregnancy takes place.

I'd been driving down a West Texas highway on my way to Marfa, the breeze blowing through my rolled-down window and Neil Young's *After the Gold Rush* on the CD player. My family originated in West Texas, but these ancestors had passed on, and all that was left of their impact were old fences and dilapidated homes. The land, however, is forever infused with their spirit, and it has always called me. I still sense them in every feature in the landscape, each desolate country road reminding me of the lives they lived and the paths they carved that would shape my existence.

As I drove over a hill in the flat terrain of the desert, I could see the vast horizon in front of me. A beam of sunlight caused my eyes to blur. I pulled over to get my focus back, and in that very moment, as I reached over to roll up the window on the passenger side, a crystal-clear vision hit me. A young brown-haired girl around the age of seven was reaching her arm out the open window of a pickup truck, driving down the highway, her fingers extended as if she were weaving the air between her fingertips. Cool evening air spilled in, and majestic sunset skies lit the backdrop. She looked over with a large yet thoughtful smile and said, "Hi, Mom."

She was speaking to *me*. I had experienced a premonition.

This visitation from the future was so powerfully real, I could not doubt it for a moment. I knew then and there that some part of my life trajectory had already been mapped out. I felt this, even at the age of 17, when I was in some ways more uncertain than I'd ever been at any other point in my life. I had just brushed elbows with my future daughter.

I realized I was sensitive to unseen forces early in my life, so this was not my first experience of "energetic" beings. I had felt them from a very young age in the form of angelic beings and Earth spirits. Children interpret the world and its mythologies through imagination. This magical realism can be the best part of childhood—it can also be overwhelming and sometimes scary, however.

After my father retired from the military when I was five, he wanted to return to spiritual work and became a Baptist missionary and preacher. My family was uprooted from the officer's quarters at an army base in Maryland to move to a small town of 2,000 in West Texas. The change was hard on everyone. I had developed very severe asthma (an affliction that is commonly known to affect people with deep psychic abilities) at age two, and the combination of environmental factors and the stress of the move exacerbated my symptoms. I spent many nights wide awake, unable to breathe and just thinking, feeling, and interpreting the empty room around me. I used the tools I was taught in Sunday school and Bible stories to navigate the darkness. I would pray to surround myself in a shield of light and recite verses commanding the "devil to get behind me." It was a crash course in sensing the forces of dark and light.

A year after the move, I woke up in the darkness to the sound of someone whispering my name. In that liminal space between waking and dreaming, I made out the shadow of a figure at the foot of my bed. I was not scared as it said to me, "Julie, do not worry or fear, there is a plan for you in this life. Rest." The next morning, I excitedly told my parents that I had been visited by an angel. They listened and believed me, but also did not make very much of it—or so I thought. Thirty years later, my father gave me a torn-out piece of paper from his journal: "May, 1984, Julie visited by angel. Told her to not worry that she had a destiny. What a special, sensitive and intuitive daughter I have. . . ." Today this note is framed on my desk, next to pictures of children I've helped shepherd onto Earth over the years. It reminds me to trust in my path.

All of these experiences were a bridge to what I consider my intuition. I experience intuition as a blended composite of thoughts, dreams, and impressions—which can be difficult to decipher. I also connect my own personal impressions with that of a universal consciousness, one that is recording the history, actions, and events of everyone on Earth. Additionally, another universal consciousness is constantly recording the psychic and energetic imprints of all sentient beings. When we ask where our visions come from, it is essential to remember that both of these mentioned records influence the answer greatly.

In seeing my future daughter, I felt I was tapping into something much larger than my mere personal knowing. And while I already knew that existence was much bigger than what I could experience with my five senses, this visitation changed everything for me. It was my first encounter from a future spirit who had not yet chosen to be born, let alone decided that it would be indelibly connected to me as my birth daughter.

It is sometimes difficult to wrap your rational mind around encountering nonmaterial energy, mostly because we look to others to determine if what we experienced was indeed "real." Much of what is determined to be real is a social agreement. Many gifted intuitives lose their voice and path due to fear of not fitting in, or even worse, persecution and judgment. Unfortunately, the intuitive wisdom that they can share is sometimes lost, and we end up in danger, as we are now, of losing our access to the universal records of wisdom, as well as intuitive and emotional intellect—all of which can empower us to advocate for not only ourselves but for our children and all other human beings.

What I have developed in my practice of spiritual fertility is teachable. And while I have honed, practiced, and perfected my own intuitive gifts over the years, what has become clear to me is that we each have the capacity to trust and cultivate intuition. The following chapters will share how to work through the traumas and filters that keep you from trusting in the unseen and energetic. And even more powerfully, I will show you how this connection has the ability to improve your fertility.

## BEYOND CONVENTIONAL MEDICINE

Almost a decade after that visit from my spirit daughter, I sat in my office in SoHo, New York City, sensing the energy of another young brown-haired girl. This time, the visitation was not for me, but for the patient lying on my treatment table. This child's spirit was also powerfully bound to her, but there were complications. Complex and difficult physical complications, which had been sustained in childhood.

After a tragic accident, which had punctured my client's lower abdomen and uterus at age eight, she was told that having children later on might be difficult and maybe even impossible. So, at 26, after a year of trying to conceive, she found me in a last-ditch effort before pursuing a surrogate. Inch by inch, we unpacked the trauma surrounding the accident—revisiting the "truths" she was told by doctors and specialists as a child and exploring how her undeveloped brain and body interpreted the events. Six months passed and she still was not pregnant, although she was healthier and happier than ever, both physically and psychologically. I asked her to keep the faith and try for just one more cycle, as I could deeply sense that her readiness was beginning to align with cosmic timing. She agreed.

At the beginning of the next cycle, her dear grandmother passed away; although sad, my client was relieved that the woman who helped care for her after her accident would no longer be in debilitating pain. Her next pregnancy test was positive. She is now the mother of four healthy and naturally conceived children. There were absolutely no complications with any of their pregnancies or births. What doctors told her would be the "truth" about her difficulty conceiving and carrying children was wrong. She found another truth that was more powerful.

As I discovered with this client, the processes of deciding to have a child, suffering from loss or infertility, or just preparing for pregnancy can create feelings of isolation and confusion. It can be challenging to turn the experience into an empowered and healthy one.

For a world that's so goal-oriented, the unseen can be a powerful tool and guide in addressing challenges around fertility. Fertility that doesn't respond to any treatment, be it conventional or holistic, is one of the hardest experiences to endure. Science cannot understand the mysteries of the womb, conception, and birth in the exact way that science cannot truly understand the beginnings of the universe. This can be puzzling and painful to experience when all that you have to comfort and explain your infertility is science.

I've worked with people passing through IVF clinics who have perfect ovarian stimulation, fertilization, and ovum growth, and yet, regardless of all laboratory test outcomes, pregnancy does not occur. One of my patients experienced three rounds of failed IVF and explained to me that she was just "the 5 percent that can't get pregnant in her age group." There was no explanation given, and no other treatment offerings except more IVF, more exploratory procedures, more genetic testing, and more of the same.

This same person, using the methods laid out in this book, rerouted this negative categorization into a positive connection with her sexuality and reproductive health. Behind her 5 percent diagnosis was a deep psychological block to becoming a mother. Beyond this deep block was a history of childhood abuse that had never been exposed— and behind the exposed abuse was a disconnect between her heart and uterus. Through all the years of fertility treatment, she never believed that she could become pregnant and had only fixated on the fact that her reproductive capacity was broken because of the shame that she carried. I learned from cases like hers that we can find solutions for fertility issues beyond the narrow confines of conventional medicine.

We need a new way to look at conception and fertility: a new way that draws from many traditions and perspectives—new and old, psychic and psychological, based in both Western and Eastern medicine—all with the purpose of supporting the healthy and spiritually integrated human of which the future Earth is in such drastic need.

## Exercise: *By Your Side*

Who in your life is by your side? Create a list of the people whom you feel are rooting for you to get to the top of the climb, and start asking them for the support you need.

Who in your life are you rooting for? Do they reciprocate the energy you share, or do they demand more than you can give? We often say "I love you" when we need to hear how much we are loved. How can you express your gratitude to those who stand with you while also fulfilling your own needs for love and support? And how can you gently start to let go of those relationships that demand more than they give?

Begin to make mental notes of how your body, heart, and mind *feel* after you spend time with co-workers, family, and friends. Imagine that your essential energy looks like a full power bar in a video game. What activities, interactions, and conversations drain your power bar the fastest? And which people, places, and rituals renew your strength? By keeping track you can better resolve to give your time and energy to the latter.

## EXPANDING BEYOND THE KNOWN

I use my intuitive skills to connect to unseen dimensions by a method that accesses what I think of as the cosmic library, making me a psychic librarian who is able to search the stacks to find the secrets hidden in even the hardest-to-find books. After I feel a strongly attached spirit in a person's energy field, I know nothing will get in that spirit's way of incarnating. The spirit will move events, meetings, energies, and encounters so that it can be born. The trick is mostly staying out of the way of the cosmic plan. Staying out of the way, but still being receptive, open, and willing to fall in love.

Surprisingly, many people are resistant to falling in love. We all can switch teams from love to fear quickly when faced with the concept of infertility. I often compare navigating infertility to war. I'm the daughter of an army colonel, so I know about war and its potential impact on the generations that follow. As a society, we now for the most part acknowledge post-traumatic stress as a real impact of war. Why do we not acknowledge the energetic battlefields of repeated miscarriage, failed IVF cycles, and negative pregnancy tests? How can we expect single individuals to fight that war alone? A war that is paramount to all else when it comes to the future of our world?

Very little of the bravery and strength needed to navigate pregnancy and birth has ever been truly recognized by our modern culture. The taboo around discussing female sexuality and anatomy, and women's monthly cycles, is still so great that one rarely hears much, if anything, about it in the media. If people can't share their unique experience with symptoms such as cramps and PMS, how can they be encouraged to disclose their battle scars and trauma from the unseen war of infertility?

Many people still bear so much judgment of those who are unable to conceive. Our beliefs, whether conscious or not, draw greatly from a kind of causal system that says you must have done something wrong to not be able to have children. Or that something must be inferior about your body, physical health, or economic status if you cannot conceive. Most people will not admit these hidden positions outright, but when you inquire just below superficial politeness, harsh indictments are not hard to find.

These pervasive opinions and belief systems are an example of energy that can influence the material world and matter. How does this hidden war impact fertility? Can unspoken judgments affect a woman's experience and fertility? We have all felt how a harbored resentment toward a spouse or partner can sabotage the relationship. Unspoken anger, sadness, and rage take real energy to maintain, and also engage the endocrine system. Stress hormones are a part of our core operating systems. They are effective and highly functional in their sworn duty to protect the animal body. And by animal body, I mean the most basic structures of what keeps us alive.

But fertility is about far more than just staying alive. Being fertile is about consciously evolving while skillfully delivering the brilliance of the genetic wisdom that came before us into an even better future. The desire to have a child can be part of this energetic upgrade. Our core curiosity in having a child relates to our own mortality and inquiry into universal principles. It's impossible to pro-create without considering the cosmos, the future of the Earth, souls, the Divine, and energy. The sense of magic that we all share in the mystery of life is our common ground. Regardless of your experience, we can all meet in this space—this neutral zone of awe, spirit, and perplexity.

The coalescence of energy that takes place before a person is conceived and born is remarkable. When making the choice to become pregnant, the mind engages in a different way than if pregnancy happens as a surprise. And if conception doesn't occur quickly, this time is typically full of countless queries as to why it is not happening for you and your partner. Here are some standard things people say about the choice in delaying trying to conceive: "There is never a perfect time," or "You are never really ready." Some standard fears are also frequently spread, such as, "You don't want to be too old," and "Childbirth is really scary and so much can go wrong."

I encourage my clients to create their own questions, based on an inventory that is far more personalized. Once these are established, we turn toward practical exercises to connect and listen to their intuitive voice and the energy before the matter. Some of those exercises will be included in this book for you to delve into on your own and with the guidance I've offered here.

As I've discovered and as I emphasize to my clients, the intuitive voice is more important than anyone else's opinion, even if that person is your partner, doctor, or loved one. The most frequent response I hear when I ask people to trust their intuition is simply that they don't know how to differentiate their intuition from fear.

This is where personal responsibility comes in. One of the reasons it is so important for all of us to consciously change the language we use (mostly unconsciously), as well as the beliefs we place around pregnancy and childbirth, is that when we infuse fear into our opinions, we make it more difficult for ourselves and those around us to connect with and trust the intuitive voice.

Fear resonates at the deepest level within our beings. It has access to the same depth of content as transgenerational trauma, which we will explore in Chapter 2. When presenting our fear to those who have not yet established their own unique set of questions and have not yet had the opportunity to develop an intuitive practice, we are essentially compromising the most powerful tool they possess. When fear is internalized, it sets off a cascade of unseen events in the hormonal body, cued by the hormone cortisol, which is meant to help us identify stress and avoid it, not to persist in living with it. These fear patterns go very deep into childhood, for most of us are taught by our parents to fear before being taught to trust ourselves.

## MOVING PAST FEAR INTO INTUITION

When I was younger, I was a rock climber. When with my best friend, Heather, as my climbing partner, I could climb up almost anything; she had an amazing belief in my ability to do so. But when climbing with others, the moment I could sense that they doubted my ability—and perhaps didn't want to see me get to the top—I would almost always falter and come down early.

Who in your life wants you to get to the top of the climb? And who does not? When approached by others who are asking for our opinions about things they should perhaps be trusting their own intuition on, how can we reframe our suggestions to support them, instead of sabotaging their climb?

It feels amazing to support someone to find and connect to what that person desires. It can also be frustrating and take time. You have to put much of your own self aside. However, what you gain is a friend or partner who is deeply connected to his or her own intuitive wisdom. This ally can similarly offer you help when you forget that you inherently know what the answers are.

I am reminded of one of my clients who came to me uncertain if and when she wanted to get pregnant. So much intuitive and energetic wisdom was present for her: a loving and healthy husband and a deep, spiritual yoga practice. She also had no material or financial concerns; she had an inheritance and was a successful yoga instructor. I inquired if she wanted to be a mother. She responded,

"Absolutely, yes, but I'm terrified by all the stories of things going wrong that I've heard from family members."

She was inundated with the belief that there was a very high chance that she would either not be able to get pregnant, or that she would have a traumatic birth. Unfortunately, the cynical culture of New York City and modern medicine tends to perpetuate worst-case scenarios. Add to this the fact that most modern mothers are exhausted, overstressed, overworked, and very undersupported. None of this was true for my well-supported and lifestyle-conscious client, but she'd still internalized the pervasive attitude of our culture around pregnancy.

I asked her to make an inventory of questions that she had and to not share these questions with anyone else, aside from me. So far, she had only picked up on the chatter around difficult, scary births, without consulting with her own inner knowing. She needed to alchemize and harness a sense of general openness to the unknown, untainted by outside influences. In this way, she could start to envision and connect to her own unique pregnancy and the spirit of her child.

Once her list was made, it included questions like: *Is my body strong enough? Am I ready to give up all the attention from my partner? I haven't had a chance to figure out what I want to do with my life—will this get in the way of my actualization?*

Her responses, when we finally got to the core, clarified that she was not ready to have a child. While she did believe she was strong enough and would someday have a healthy baby, she was being intuitively called to work on her own spiritual path a bit longer. She felt guilty for being "selfish," as her partner was ready and so many of the circumstances in her life were perfect for starting a family.

She knew she wasn't ready on an intuitive level, however, and her guilt drove her to latch on to negative thoughts and opinions about childbirth, which offered her a "valid" excuse not to get pregnant.

The potential consequences of this misplaced reasoning might have been dire in the long run and far worse than just admitting what she wanted. It was important for her to see that she didn't have to align her fertility with these fearful excuses; instead, she could make the empowered choice to pursue her own path. For the time being, she made the decision to follow her intuition and rule out the strong beliefs and needs of those around her. Weeks after our meeting, she received an invitation to travel to Africa and run a nonprofit volunteer organization dear to her heart.

My client's story is a perfect example of how it takes practice to connect with what is intuitively true for us. Sometimes, it is difficult to differentiate fear from intuition because, sometimes, fear is the very thing we are using to block ourselves from our intuitive knowing. Fear is the excuse we fall back on to avoid connecting to what we already know, especially if that information feels disruptive or threatening—or if it is in conflict with what we think we *should* want or what others want from us. The truth is, it is always hard to be the first person to raise your hand to state that something is not right. But far more painful than speaking up for a core belief is living with a situation that grates against your soul and creates self-doubt and distrust. Advocacy for your current and future children begins with advocacy for your intuitive connection and voice.

## Exercise: *Intuition Inventory*

Sometimes it is difficult to differentiate fear from intuition because sometimes fear is the very thing we are using to block ourselves from our intuitive knowing. Create an inventory of questions that describe your intuition, fears, and beliefs about your fertility and becoming a mother. To help you determine these questions, imagine yourself freely and privately conversing with a great mystic who has the power to see into the future, but is also able to hold you in a nonjudgmental space without being invested in an outcome. I call this force the oracle.

The oracle is a reflection of your unconscious, your intuition, and your higher self. When you give voice to the questions that are difficult to say out loud or to write down, like the ones my client shared in this chapter, a pathway of energy is created that will help you find the answers you are looking for. Often, in order to receive guidance and help, we simply need to ask a question. Set a timer for 10 minutes and start writing your list of questions. If you're not finished when the timer goes off, keep writing until you're done.

## SPIRITUAL ADVOCACY

Most of my clients are more than ready to become pregnant. Many have sensed the energy of their future children, and their intuition and desire are present. I have mentioned that this book is informed by my clients, mostly women, and my desire to document their unseen battles and the strength of spirit they mustered to traverse it. While part of my job is to relentlessly support my clients in developing and trusting their intuition, I'm also an advocate for the spirits of their children, sometimes before my clients are even aware of the attachments.

This can be hard for my clients, and they sometimes feel inadequate or jealous that I can experience connections they cannot. The nature of the work of spiritual fertility is to recognize that we are all collectively united, much more than our rational world lets us express. There is a deeper intelligence orchestrating the events of our lives and those we will meet on our life path. And just as I play a role in their destiny, they do in mine. With time, self-care, and by removing the filters that obstruct the connection to their intuition, everyone can feel the unseen connections of energy.

What I sense in a session is a reflection of what each client has present within her. Connections are often clearer to me than they are to my clients because I am a neutral observer. One of my clients, whom I will call Diana, brought her youngest daughter with her to a session. I could instantly feel the immense depth of observation and psychic abilities this little girl possessed. I encouraged her to come to the session, because I was very aware of how she was dominating the energetic field of her mother. There was nothing negative about her presence, but her needs were so strong that her mother was unable to be completely available. As a result, I was unable to get a clear read of the mother with the two-year-old's energy manifesting so strongly.

Diana had experienced a miscarriage recently and was confused and scared as to why it had happened. I would like to take a moment here to address a topic that we will explore in depth later in Chapter 2. Miscarriages are never caused by negative energy, karmic forces, or in this case, an older sibling. Many people fear that they have done something wrong or encountered bad energy to make a miscarriage happen. This is incorrect. Miscarriages are always and completely a matter of timing. And just as one can fall deeply and completely in love with a person only to realize the timing for a relationship or deeper commitment isn't right, so too, the timing of conception and pregnancy might simply not be right. Love streams beyond what we know or can control. Timing is similar, and as much as we think we can control it, most of it happens on God's watch.

So, when Diana told me that after our session together her little girl would not stop asking questions about me—such as when she could see me again and if I could be her mommy—I knew that our session was not about my client's desire to get pregnant again. Advocating for a child's spirit can extend to not only those children who have yet to be born, but also to those who are already here. I've seen many pathways for pregnancy open when the energetic needs of siblings were addressed. We will discuss later in Chapter 9 the soul contracts between parents, unborn children, and their siblings, and how they impact fertility.

I asked Diana about the circumstances around her daughter's conception and pregnancy, and if there had been anything particularly dangerous about it. Yes, she said resoundingly, screening had shown that the baby was carrying some dangerous genetic variations that could result in developmental and physical delays and disease. Much of this child's experience in utero was veiled in her parents' energy of wondering if she was going to even make it—and if she did, whether she would be healthy.

So, when she was born healthy, strong, and cognitively perfect, everyone exhaled, relaxed, and went about life as if nothing had happened. But the initial energetic imprint of fear was still with the young girl, confirming the vigilance I had felt so strongly from her, as she had been so closely watched and monitored pre-birth.

Two things happened after I learned this information about Diana's daughter. First, we addressed and cleared my client's unconscious beliefs and fear of being the cause of her daughter's genetic variations. In addition, we cleared the residual trauma from her daughter's field by bringing awareness to it and creating a ritual that her entire family participated in. In doing so, we looked directly at the energetic elephant in the room and healed the unconscious holding patterns around both the mother and daughter. *Clearing* is a general term that I use to describe this process of how an unresolved issue or event is identified and resolved through a healing process. In this instance, we also cleared my client's sense that the recent miscarriage was somehow connected to her earlier pregnancy.

## THE HEALING CONNECTION

I have seen time and time again the power of working on the psychic level within fertility, and its positive impact on healing trauma from this lifetime and others. Interestingly, as deep as this work goes in revisiting the darkest blame, shame, and guilt, most people can move seamlessly through clearing it once it has been identified. The energetic help from the other side, via the spirit of the child who is coming home, provides a healing connection, one full of joy and vitality.

We often look at children as separate wards or responsibilities, or as extensions of our own beings. But when we acknowledge that they, too, are sovereign in their energetics, we begin a different conversation. This conversation acknowledges the power of the unseen and the connectivity of the material world and the spiritual world. Strengthening that spiritual connection provides guidance and clarity when you are faced with challenges. Every challenge you meet in life has the potential to help break you open and promote evolution. Creating a spiritual path within fertility balances the hormonal and nervous systems and promotes happiness and well-being—while also helping you get pregnant.

Emotional maturity plays a tremendous role in understanding and working with energy. Being responsible for your own psychic space while practicing the type of self-care that is necessary for you to connect with your intuition requires emotional discipline. I am not suggesting that you suppress your emotions, but instead gain perspective on how your emotions can inform the psychic connection with your child's spirit.

Emotion is sometimes a dirty word in this world, where being in control is the cultural default. Emotions serve as messengers and act as liaisons between our bodies and the environment. Think of the times that you have felt something before you could analyze it, or express it in words. Emotions are the energy before the matter. They serve as direct translators for our nervous system and hormonal bodies, and protect us in times when threats and traumas from the environment occur so quickly that our rational minds can't process and react fast enough.

And yet, to be perceived as a highly emotional person—more specifically, a highly emotional woman—is still judged in our society instead of praised. But we can begin to access our emotions as an aid in our process. Emotional intelligence is a skill that can be studied and learned, just like analytic wisdom. And in many cases, a keen emotional intelligence is what we admire in our friends and family members. Individuals who have taken the time to learn their own emotional landscape are typically powerhouses of clarity. They act fluidly and with confidence, even in the most stressful of situations.

What is it within each of us that keeps us from expressing our emotional experience with honesty? How can we learn to become acquainted with our most difficult feelings, so that we might better understand and recognize messages from our deepest depths as they drift into our daily lives?

Ancient temples and churches followed a clear and methodical orientation. They are often built to model the heavens, and are arranged in accord with the compass directions. These foundations create the space for a higher-level connection between self and the spirit. Sacred spaces are meant to inspire a life in which humanity reflects the holy. If you are yearning for inspiration and clarity as to what to do next on your path through fertility, the answer may be as simple as returning to essential self-care and emotional maturity.

Remember that your body is also a sacred space, and determine the pillars of what you absolutely need in order to support the structure of your spirit. Do not compromise when it comes to integrating these supportive pillars into your life. Most of the subtle energetics that are working behind the scenes become clear when you listen to what essentially gives you happiness and health. Consider the times in your life when you have felt the most connected, happy in your body, relaxed in your nervous system, and in love with life. Identifying and incorporating into your daily life the tools that helped you obtain this balance is essential as you do the work of this book.

## Spiritual Fertility Essentials

In this chapter, we began looking at your relationship to intuition as an ally in the journey to motherhood. Examining what you think is "true" about your spiritual and physical health provides insight into areas of your life where you need support and healing. Creating an inventory of your own unique questions about fertility will provide you with the clarity needed to reestablish and reconnect to your intuitive wisdom and practice. The first step in finding the new energy of your child's spirit is to acknowledge the energies at work in your life. Focusing on yourself and the people in your life who support and lift your spirit up is essential to your well-being. Learning to ask for help from your support system is a powerful tool and an essential practice to carry into pregnancy and motherhood.

# Chapter 2

# Transgenerational Trauma and the Trauma Surrounding Our Births

We are individually and collectively influenced by the traumatic events of our lifetimes. Major catastrophes such as war, displacement from home, childhood abuse, and random acts of violence create reverberations and ripple effects in our lives that impact how we view ourselves and others. These impressions are also handed down from generation to generation, manifesting as information that gets lodged in our nervous systems and compels our behavior in mysterious ways. However, investigating trauma can offer us powerful touch points for healing, and for simply joining with the collective fear of our fellow human beings with the utmost empathy.

Perhaps you have not been personally affected by a traumatic event in this lifetime, but chances are someone in your family line has. Trauma is an ancient concept, originating from the Greek word for *wound*. Wounds can injure our physical, psychological, and emotional bodies—and while we can heal from many wounds, some remain open and raw for a long time. Such is the case in the unhealed wounds we inherit from our ancestors, as well as the trauma from our own perinatal and birth experiences that can be passed from one generation to the next—in some cases, even influencing our fertility.

There is significant research on how those who survived extreme physical and mental trauma, starvation, and abuse passed on a heightened nervous system, endocrine sensitivity, hyper-inflammatory conditions, and reproductive imbalance to their children. Hypervigilance, naturally developed in times of strife, particularly impacts fertility. Currently, the Middle East has one of the highest male factor infertility rates on the planet, most of which can be attributed to the stress and impact of war over the last several decades. The legacy of transgenerational trauma is such that even if universal peace were declared tomorrow, generations to come could still be adversely affected by the wars of the past.

Trauma need not be as extreme as war or genocide to be harmful and inheritable—small and overlooked daily traumas such as poverty and domestic abuse are just as injurious. The microtraumas in an individual's life span can also accumulate into more established currents that direct the flow of a person's life. Happily, there is a way to heal these wounds and change the future.

Each time we choose to have a child, we are presented with the opportunity to reframe our individual histories, and by extension, our familial line. Herein lies one of the earliest and most significant gifts that our children offer us: the ability to reflect on what has not worked and to move forward to a new model of the family. Infertility can feel isolating, unfair, and painful, doubly so when much of the contributing trauma was handed to us by our ancestors, who might not have put in the healing work necessary. There is a concept in holistic medicine suggesting that a symptom that is not resolved will linger under the surface for years until it again finds an opportunity to express itself in hopes of being fixed. Applying this to transgenerational trauma suggests that even if you do achieve pregnancy with ease, you and your children will at some time have to resolve the unfinished business of your lineage. In consciously conceiving you get to set the time for this healing and get to do it on your watch. This resolution is profound and not only helps you get pregnant, but also enables you to be fully present for the joy of being a mother.

## HOW TRAUMA INFLUENCES OUR REPRODUCTIVE CAPACITY

While studying obstetrics in Shanghai, one of the most impressive and apparent differences from the United States that I observed in the labor and delivery room was the temperature: It was hot. Really hot. In general, China is exceedingly sparing with its use of energy. I recall graciously being invited over to one of the doctor's homes for dinner one evening and being quite surprised to see my host answer the door in a full-length winter jacket. We all sat around the table in cold-weather garb while feasting on her family's favorite recipes. So this was unusual.

"Why is it kept so warm in the delivery room?" I asked the doctor.

"Cold is the first trauma," she replied, "so we try to make it warm to ensure that babies and their mamas have less trauma."

The doctor understood one of the essential aspects of our humanity: our mastery of fire and our ability to rise above the elements. When exposed to cold, our muscles and bodies tense and we withdraw from the environment. Our respiration quickens, we begin to shiver, and we might reserve energy by lowering and saving our voice. We also conserve energy by slowing our digestion. Depending on the length and location of exposure to cold, the impact can remain with the body for a lifetime.

In my childhood, I recall always being puzzled as to why my father, a seemingly tall and robust ex–Army Ranger, still needed extra blankets on his legs and feet at night.

"Service to the nation," he would explain to me when I asked why. It was not until sometime later that I learned the effects of frostbite; cold exposure even at the young age of 21 could linger in his body forever. You see, some traumas are so intense that even briefly witnessing them can leave behind a residue. It is difficult to erase such experiences from memory, even when we are not fully conscious of them. However, the faster the injury is addressed, named, contained, and processed, the less likely it is to have long-lasting—and fertility-impacting—results.

Thus, it is that postpartum care in China that greatly supports the essential energetic environment of the mother by paying close attention to avoiding cold, maintaining warmth, eating warm foods, and obtaining plenty of rest. There is a cultural understanding that the degree of care for the mother and baby at the time of the delivery and during the postpartum period impacts future fertility.

In contrast, Western medical intervention and its extreme methodology can interfere with several natural processes that occur at birth. For instance, without dilation of the cervical canal, women cannot produce oxytocin, considered the "love and bonding" hormone. Without its presence, mothers find it hard to connect and relate to their babies. Breastfeeding also produces oxytocin—so when mothers do not breastfeed their children, oxytocin is not sufficiently produced in their body.

Along the same lines, an orthopedic surgeon friend of mine now uses a heated blanket to warm the body and muscles of his patients before surgery. This positively influences the outcome by encouraging tight muscles to relax instead of constrict. Adding heat might seem like an obvious and straightforward way to combat trauma and positively impact health, but sometimes the most obvious solution is the hardest to see. The outcome of surgery can change when we merely add a warm blanket. And with this, the plausibility of trauma—often considered a default experience, given the ubiquitous nature of human suffering—is substantially reduced.

## THE SUBTLE WOUNDS OF
## TRANSGENERATIONAL TRAUMA

Factors such as severe cold or surgical trauma might be more obvious than the more subtle wounds of inherited beliefs and patterns. My work includes identifying potential ways unresolved injuries are passed down from one generation to the next (transgenerational trauma), and how these might interfere with fertility. I do this by listening for specific key phrases and descriptions from my patients. Frequently, people know they are carrying a psychic or emotional burden for their family. They often talk about feeling very different from their siblings and other family members, and how they either walk away from conflict within their family or avoid direct contact with them altogether.

If you intuitively feel like transgenerational trauma might be playing a role in your ability to get pregnant, there are several ways to begin to reflect and create an inventory of what might be happening behind the scenes. The following are some—but not all—of the most common factors that I look for in my one-on-one work with clients:

- Relatives who lived or died in concentration camps or as prisoners of war, or who were victims of acts of terror

- Family secrets, either spoken or unspoken, such as incest, physical or verbal abuse, disease, or psychiatric confinement

- Being born to replace or fix the grief from the loss of a child or other family member

- Adoption, undisclosed use of reproductive technologies such as donor egg or sperm, being born from secret or scandalous events such as affairs

- Death of a parent at a formative age

- Medical histories, especially on the matriarchal line, of miscarriage and stillbirth

We will explore several of these concepts throughout the book, as they often relate to the ecosystem of fertility. To begin, let's look at some of the more common themes of inherited trauma.

## TRAUMA THROUGH THE FAMILY LINE

Many people grow up believing that the stories of chronic miscarriage, traumatic births, and infertility they hear from mothers, aunts, and friends will undoubtedly be what they experience. This is doubly true about transgenerational myths of fertility. The stories that people hear from childhood into adulthood influence how they understand and connect to their sexuality and to their reproductive capacity. Take, for instance, the second child of Diana, the client we spoke about in Chapter 1. Her narrative could have been influenced by a mother who had not healed and a lingering psychological darkness over her own birth, which had already been traumatic due to the emergency C-section.

Sometimes, within a family, individuals are stigmatized or scapegoated for being too sensitive or demanding too much attention. While this may seem specific to the personalities involved, it might actually point to a pattern perpetuated through the family line, or a belief cemented and repeated from generation to generation. If this is the case, someone may be making visible the symptoms of a deeper and older trauma in the family. It's painful to listen to the whistleblowers of a family, especially when there is little or no time to process their revelations or when they have been labeled mentally ill, but they can air many uncomfortable and necessary truths about our family trauma.

Even the way we are taught to listen is often directly inherited from the structures we observe in our formative years. Did someone hold space for you to speak as a child? Or were your words and ideas immediately shut down?

Half of the battle with understanding both transgenerational trauma and trauma from our own births is in identifying and naming it. The act of holding space for individuals to express their intuitive hits without judgment or quick dismissal typically exposes many of the most common reasons they are labeled as disruptive to the family. This may include the individual's reluctance to speak; an overreliance on rationalism; a penchant for cynicism; and overly exaggerated responses of anger, sadness, and the like. These all need to be addressed for someone to heal from trauma.

Ironically, sometimes the most secretive traumas can be the most apparent because people seem to go out of their way to avoid them and never speak of them. Family secrets can encompass a wide variety of topics—from mental illness and institutionalization to disease, imprisonment, adultery, adoption, illegitimacy, financial ruin, and abandonment. In modern times, extensive reproductive medical treatments, and making the choice to never disclose their use to the resulting children, can also contribute to another type of family secret. This is one that ultimately can injure everyone, especially the child who might later face his or her own reproductive difficulties, seemingly without cause.

Interestingly, people who try the hardest to keep the secrets close and hidden are typically the ones who have the most amounts of shame and guilt around the trauma. It only takes one curious whistleblower to awkwardly out the information that has been so well kept for generations—but that person is often met with the most voluble ridicule, and sometimes with exile. In particular, hidden information about children born in secretive ways—such as out of wedlock, as the result of extensive fertility struggles and treatments, from an affair, or during times of extreme fear or abuse—can energetically encode that child with a sense of not belonging, or of difference. Sometimes, this realization comes to an absolute head when a person who voices (or represents) the family's private world decides to have her own children and comes face-to-face with the undercover records she is holding.

## PATTERNS OF TRAUMA

I frequently observe patterns of trauma that can correspond to dates and seasons within a family's history. For instance, one of my patients, whom I will call Shayla, initially came to see me because she was concerned about a pattern she perceived around miscarriages she'd had over the years, all of which had occurred in October. While she had successfully carried two pregnancies, she subsequently experienced two separate miscarriages that both occurred at different stages of her pregnancy. The first miscarriage took place at 7 weeks, and the second at 13.

Shayla explained that she felt cursed and was now terrified to be pregnant during the month of October.

Sometimes it is difficult to determine if an event like this, which has an element of cyclical timing, is caused by transgenerational trauma or if it is a type of "new" trauma that might be passed down if it is not healed. In Shayla's case, I suggested that we do a timeline exercise (see sidebar on page 35) that I often use to determine events that have majorly impacted health. Starting with the present moment and working backward, I encouraged her to record significant life events, both positive and negative. These can include such things as loss of a job, death of a family member, marriage, birth, illness, car accidents, etc.

It is surprising how many of our major events can quickly pass by without our acknowledging the significant impact they have on our life's course. Such was the case with Shayla. She had not realized the correlation between the birth of her second daughter in the month of October and the two miscarriages. She listed intense delivery as an important life occurrence, six years before her first miscarriage.

As I asked extensive questions about what she experienced, Shayla went on to describe an extremely dangerous birth for both herself and her daughter. The pregnancy had been healthy up until the last two weeks, when she began to experience severe and painful cramps. Her doctors chose to induce early, a decision that Shayla did not agree with but felt pressured into. The labor did not progress, and an emergency C-section was performed, during which my patient's heart rate, as well as the baby's, dipped dramatically. Shayla was stabilized, but her child spent three weeks in the NICU (neonatal intensive care unit), during which time Shayla's father, who had been in good health, suddenly passed away. My patient had to decide between leaving her newborn at the hospital alone, caring for a small child, and traveling to attend her dad's funeral. She chose not to attend the funeral, which would require her to fly across the country—a decision that she later came to regret.

"Do you intuitively feel there is a connection between the life events that occurred around the birth of your daughter in October and the miscarriages?" I asked.

"I do," she responded, "but I am afraid to admit it because I don't feel there is anything I can do to fix it. And if I can't fix it, it means that I will continue to have miscarriages. I really loved my father dearly, and not being able to say goodbye has haunted me."

Herein lies a window into a deep unconscious and unseen inheritance that can perpetuate trauma from one generation to the next. For Shayla, so many associations with sadness, loss, and grief in the month of October—her daughter's birth month—could impact her daughter's own psychic and energetic realms, imprinting her with a type of secondary trauma that contributes to her own personal narrative about fertility.

It's important to acknowledge here that people can also rush into pregnancy to try to quickly fix an emptiness typically felt in the wake of loss or death. Processing loss can take time, and even when you feel like your mind has integrated the shock and you can move forward, your heart and body might be working on a different timeline of healing. When maternal age and pregnancy are added to the process of healing from grief and loss, the added pressure to quickly conceive can add to both the recovery process and the time it can take to become pregnant. Such was the case with Shayla, whose heartbreak exponentially increased with each loss.

The practical magic that ultimately helped this client conceive and carry to term was not found in supplements, hormonal panels, complex procedures, or IVF, but in allowing her original injuries to heal with time, space, and self-reflection. Shayla traveled to her father's grave in October and with the help of her husband and children, restaged the funeral she had missed. The process uncovered a well of grief that she had not known she was carrying. Her healing allowed her to reframe her trauma into gratitude, not only for her deceased father but also for the spirits of the two children she had lost. In looking back, she believed that these miscarriages had been her greatest teachers—and while she would always hold them close to her heart, she understood their more significant meaning in the chain of her life and that of her family's.

Her third child, who was due October 21, was born via VBAC, or vaginal birth after cesarean, on November 1. Shayla had successfully moved beyond the pattern.

If you are aware that the energy and environment leading up to a child's birth is particularly stressful and intense, special care and consciousness should be taken to acknowledge the presence of that child's spirit. I like to direct my clients to imagine that their unborn child is just like a cartoon angel sitting on their shoulder, listening and observing the events that are unfolding. We are human, after all, and because being human is difficult, you don't have to be perfect. Simple awareness and recognition are enough to make all the difference. It is especially important to ensure that a child's spirit is met with a unique and inviting welcome, not an imposed expectation that the child will fix heartbreak, relational disconnect, loss, or depression.

## Exercise: *The Timeline*

Stretch a long piece of paper across a table, counter, wall, or desk. Draw a long straight line across the middle from left to right. In the middle of this line, mark the day and time of your birth. Everything before this point of your birth is the timeline of the energetic matrix that you came from, and the events after this point reflect the major events in your life. Add positive events, such as falling in love or graduating from college, above the line. Add negative events, such as childhood illness or a disruptive family move, below the line.

Starting with the present moment, represented at the end of the line, and working backward, begin to record significant life events, both positive and negative, from your own lifetime. Work backward toward your birth and record what you know about your birth, including your gestation and conception. Once you have reached your birth date, begin to record what you know of your family line, paying special attention to topics that were covered in this chapter. This is also an intuitive exercise, meaning that you can write down any thoughts, feelings, or intuitive "hits" that you believe are relative, even if they do not make sense to your rational mind. Gaining awareness of these events will shed light on your current fertility journey. It is surprising how many of our major events can quickly pass by without our acknowledging the significant impact they have on our life's course.

## THE IMPACT OF IVF AND BIRTH
## TRAUMA ON YOUR FERTILITY

Many traditions of medicine and bodywork take into account the type of birth you had as a causal factor that impacts your health. Specific physical postures can be the effect of how you lay in the womb, and holding patterns of tension in the body might be the result of being born breech or via forceps or suction.

If your birth process was interrupted at a stage of labor, such as during transition as you were moving through the cervical canal, some traditions hold you will always have difficulty with transitions in life. Essentially, birth can be a refractive mirror of transgenerational trauma and a precursor or predictor of how your earliest experience in the world might impact the rest of your life. Here are some major themes to look for that indicate trauma around your own birth (note, many of these are experienced at a higher rate among children born via the use of reproductive medicine):

- C-section birth

- The presence and use of forceps or suction to extract you from the birth canal

- Premature birth

- Induction based on being over due date

- Separation from parents immediately after birth

- Death of mother in childbirth or in the postpartum period

Many of the repetitive traumas around inherited reproductive difficulties are seen in the story of a person's conception and birth. I ask each of my patients what they know of their own conceptions and births—and if they don't know anything, I encourage them to learn more from their family. Inquiring for potentially traumatic stories can be dangerous. It is important to hold space and boundaries, so as to be able to listen and learn without allowing the discovery to impact you too much. I suggest going into such conversations with an extremely open mind, recording them if possible and making the questions concise and succinct. I've included an exercise on page 15 that will help you take an intuitive inventory. The answers that you will find in this inventory will typically give you the first clue to potential trauma influencing fertility.

Some of the less-navigated topics around conception and birth, even among those within the world of fertility medicine, include the energetics of embryo extraction and storage. (I differentiate this from egg freezing, where the egg has not been fertilized.) I once had a conversation with a young woman in her 20s that struck me as revelatory. When she asked me what I did and I shared with her that I was a fertility specialist, she responded as no one ever had. "Do you think that being born from IVF has lifelong complications?" A little puzzled, I inquired if she was working on a research paper for school. "I was born via IVF," she stated, "and I've always felt that the cognitive difficulties I have are related to the way I was conceived, but no one believes me."

One of the most injurious traumas that can impact a person's ability to trust her intuition—and to a larger extent, her life path—is using science or medical facts to mitigate her instinct and experience. It is important to listen and not overinterpret someone's views, no matter how factual you find them to be. "It could be," I responded, and we went on to speak for a while about her story and how it might impact her fertility. I shared with her how some children can recall past lives and can give specific details about who, where, and when they lived—and how some children who shared a womb with a twin that did not make it to birth can exhibit a noticeable absence of that twin.

I've observed that some children express loss or sadness over what they describe as leaving their brothers and sisters behind: Their parents can become confused by their grief because they often did not have siblings. More in-depth inquiry typically uncovers that these children were born from IVF, and that there were other stored embryos from the same fertilization and extraction. While this might sound impossible, when it comes to the energetics of conception we can only hypothesize about how an individual becomes an individual, and when consciousness becomes embodied.

The process of IVF is challenging to navigate, and I've found that my patients who voice concern over these other frozen potential children soon become too overwhelmed with the process and the end goal of becoming pregnant. And because the stress of living in the modern world is enormous and demands so much from each of us, it can be hard to find the time to be reflective about a topic such as the secret life of frozen embryos and what consciousness they may or may not have.

Many people have initial resistance and fear around returning to the memory of the IVF process and even more opposition to the acknowledgment that they—who often wanted children so badly that they were willing to endure intense fertility treatments—could somehow potentially be leaving other children behind in cold storage. Some women I have worked with state that they never want to do IVF again because, to them, it felt as difficult as a miscarriage or an abortion.

None of this is spoken about in public, and typically remains in an individual's internal dialogue. However, a guiding principle of spiritual fertility is to shed light onto the places that elicit the emotions of blame, shame, and guilt. To destigmatize the shame of IVF, we must allow it to be spoken about and acknowledged as what it is: an intense life event. To mitigate the guilt of leaving embryos behind, we must celebrate their sacrifice for the life of the child who did make it. Lastly, to move on and heal energetically at a societal level, we must resolve the blame that we show ourselves and our fellow human beings for needing assisted reproductive medicine in the first place.

## BEING MINDFUL OF TRAUMA WHILE APPROACHING CONCEPTION

It is my intention that approaching the conception and birth of your children through the practices that this book teaches can help you overwrite transgenerational narratives and promote conscious conception, which takes into account the mind, body, and spiritual connections.

There is an unseen intelligence at work when it comes to conception, pregnancy, and birth. Trusting in this intelligence and in your body's own intuition is essential to deterring the factors that might be interfering with its natural progression. As you remove the filters of trauma and stress, new unwanted energetics that enter into your environment will become clearer, and you will know how to block them from impacting your fertility.

Such was the case for my patient, Rachel, who learned how to deflect jealousy and envy from her sister, who was harming her connection to the fertility process. Rachel's family had a rough history; her great-grandmother had escaped a concentration camp that took the lives of her entire family. This woman married the man who helped her survive and moved to America, where the severe starvation that she had suffered significantly influenced her reproductive health.

Rachel's grandmother was a miracle child, born after many miscarriages and years of failed pregnancy attempts. Rachel's own mother had not experienced fertility issues and was able to conceive and carry three healthy children to term. Unfortunately, because the transgenerational trauma was never addressed, that pattern of infertility persisted. Rachel's older sister went through several failed rounds of IVF and intrauterine insemination (IUI), and was devastated by the failures. So, when Rachel and her husband decided to start their family, Rachel was understandably concerned and expressed anxiety and fear about her own ability to conceive.

What Rachel *did* have working for her was a keen curiosity and an openness to healing; these two powerful tools, combined with trusting her gut, led her to me and the methods of this book. We set out to work immediately on helping her to establish clear boundaries when communicating with her family, especially her sister.

I'd like to take a moment to address how, when women start to set boundaries, they often can experience guilt and shame for what they feel is a type of selfishness. It is not easy to prioritize your own emotional and physical needs, but this is essential for healing. Sometimes expressing transgenerational trauma for a family is the result of a soul contract we have made to take on the pain and ultimately heal it for those who came before us. The significant point, which I made to Rachel, was that when it comes to transgenerational healing, everything she did to mend the inherited wounds was working reflexively to also heal the wounds of the past. This meant that the clearer her boundaries and the more loyalty she had to herself, the deeper and more accessible the healing would be for her sister, as well. Rachel understood, but she needed some major energetic backup when coming face-to-face with her family, and she got just that in the exercise that I call the Golden Passport (see sidebar on page 43).

Later in this book we will discuss the importance of language and belief systems around fertility. While you will find this exercise relevant within the context of that section, I encourage you to use any of these practical magic exercises whenever they may be helpful. Remember, one of the guiding principles of spiritual fertility is trusting yourself and your intuition *above all others*. That said, the Golden Passport is an extremely useful therapeutic tool for almost any situation. It has its roots in the ancient energy medicine of *qigong,* which cultivates an internal warmth and energy that, when called upon, acts as a psychic immune system.

Years ago, to empower one of my patients to enforce boundaries, I printed up a mock passport made of gold paper and handed it to her, explaining that it was the ultimate pass that would take her out of any place, conversation, situation, or bad vibe that she came across. The Golden Passport meant she did not have to explain or justify her departure; she could merely exit the situation without a word. It worked like a charm!

I began to give these "passports" to my most energetically empathetic and susceptible clients, always with the instruction that it symbolized they could just walk away from any trigger that they knew might impact their fertility. Society teaches that it is rude to leave a conversation without a reason, but from the vantage point of spiritual fertility, your spiritual and energetic health trumps good manners.

Our family members, who have the opportunity to love and support us more than anyone, in particular tend to keep a running ledger of what they might call our selfish acts and disrespects. For those of you whose softer voices tend to be deafened by the louder ones, it is especially empowering to realize there is absolutely nothing wrong with simply leaving a toxic situation. As the Golden Passport never expires, you will be able to use it again and again, well past conception, pregnancy, and childbirth.

Consciousness is one of the most critical techniques you can bring into the fertility process when you are aware that family trauma negatively affects you. Merely cultivating a daily practice—such as a walk or meditation in which you allow yourself to acknowledge and hear your internal dialogue without blame, shame, and guilt—can provide a more transparent perspective into who and what in your environment enforces these impulses instead of helping you mitigate the stress.

**Exercise:** *The Golden Passport*

Make a golden passport for yourself. Create a document, preferably on golden or yellow paper, that will fit inside your wallet. Write your name and date of birth on the passport, as well as the statement: "Never Expires." As you start to work with how the energetics of your environment impact you and your fertility, begin to freely use this golden passport as the ultimate pass out of any place, conversation, situation, or bad vibe that you come across. When you use the Golden Passport, you do not have to explain or justify your departure; you can merely exit the situation without a word.

## HEALING ANCESTRAL LINES

When we consider the energy surrounding the issue of fertility, we are able to look at the larger picture of how we fit within our lineage. Imagine everyone on Earth has chosen to be here. Assume that the family line you were born into was resonant with an aspect of your eternal soul, regardless of the pain, arguments, and disconnects you may have encountered. Just like a bee to a flower, you too were attracted to land when and where you did.

I like to compare preparing for conception to planting bushes and plants that attract butterflies. How could a beautiful creature hatched from a cocoon thousands of miles away find its way over mountains, rivers, and streams into your yard—and even more amazingly, into your gaze? So many things are orchestrated behind the scenes for that moment to occur, which all began with your intent to call in a butterfly. Even if you just planted the shrub nonchalantly, knowing that butterflies would find it, you still participated in impacting the energetics. The magical moment of this viewing, as your intent comes into creation, can bring deep peace and connection to the larger forces that unify us all as humans. When we become conscious of what we are doing, our impact becomes more meaningful and perhaps less destructive. Indeed, while the moment of awe when you first hold your newborn child is indescribable in so many ways, those emotions are often compared to a sense of peace in a higher plan that is at work in the universe.

However, it is not enough to treat conception and fertility with the deepest reverence. To create a comfortable landing place for our future children, we must understand our trauma responses on a deeper and subtler level. The ways in which we allow trauma to be embedded in our systems can have far-reaching effects. The impact one life can have is significant in ways that cannot be understood. Choices that we make in our communities represent the culture and history of all the people who live there, and who ever lived there in the past. Small traumas impact how people behave.

I recently noticed that I avoided a particular street in my neighborhood of Brooklyn.

*Why don't I ever walk down that road?* I asked myself, only to instantly remember witnessing a violent act there over a decade earlier. Just as we all avoid specific paths that have been imprinted with negative and painful memories, these individual avoidances can exponentially influence the direction our family, community, and ultimately, the world will take.

This is also my experience with how fertility is currently practiced. Many people, supported by the medical system, take action to avoid pathways that are embedded with the memory of trauma. There is a collective default to rely on science and rationalism, especially when faced with fear of the unknown. But one thing is for sure: We are a product not only of the generations that came before us, but also of the lives that our ancestors lived, the environments in which they existed, and the people with whom they chose to merge. While science will someday support this statement with universally agreed-on facts, we already have concrete proof of the impact and effects of our environment on our individual bodies.

At a dinner party, I once sat next to a very interesting mother of two. She described herself as the child of two extremely rational New York City doctors and as a feminist and an author.

"What do you do?" she asked, curious. Usually, I answer that I'm a holistic fertility doctor and medical intuitive, but that night, I was feeling especially open and relaxed.

"I have the gift of sensing the spirits of unborn babies, and I help people connect and conceive."

"Wow," she responded, "like a psychic?"

"Yes, like a psychic, but more like an advocate of the intuitive," I replied.

We continued to speak of the mystery of pregnancy and birth and the magic of the unknown. I often experience when talking with people who claim to be extraordinarily analytical and "anti-woo-woo" that they open up and share radically nonrational stories of dreams, visions, and energetic awareness of their child's spirit prior to birth. I'm always so pleased to hear the staunchest skeptics admit that when it comes to their children and their love for them, something that is impossible to understand via the rational mind kicks in. As I began to explain how I first experienced my gifts, with the story of my daughter's appearance in my energetic field that I shared in Chapter 1, her brow furrowed with what I thought was a skeptical intent. Much to my surprise, however, she exclaimed, "I can make sense of the presence of babies' spirits and the way that the transgenerational trauma that you are describing can impact fertility because I know that we, as women, carry all of the eggs that might turn into children in our ovaries even before we are born. So, my daughter's potential children, my future grandchildren, were actually living inside me for a small period of time."

"Exactly! You were in your grandmother's womb just as I was in my grandmother's womb."

She was referring to the fact that women, unlike men (who continuously generate new sperm), develop our ovarian reserve around week 20 of our gestation, shoring up the direct lineage and connection to the past and giving reason to an otherwise hidden knowledge. My new friend had powerfully connected the tools of the spirit with those of modern scientific knowledge. Her curiosity and openness beautifully linked together what so many women I work with intuitively understand: the female body is an archive, and its halls of wisdom extend deeply into the history of the planet.

Intuitive knowledge can be very difficult to defend in the analytical world. But in the end, as the filters of trauma are cleared, your unique and individual wisdom will be undeniable. As the world becomes more and more diverse, the homogeneous religious, moral, and cultural standards that at one point provided a more consistently agreed-upon narrative (at least for people with privilege and power) are becoming less and less relevant. I've mentioned the great window of opportunity for healing that occurs when choosing to become a parent. At that point, many of the ruts and patterns that we repeat from previous histories have a chance to be addressed and cleared so they will not be passed on to future generations. Infertility is a symptom of a deeper wound that must be treated to heal completely.

Often, people think that if they just have a successful pregnancy and healthy child, all the pain and hurt of the past will lift. For some this is true, but the patterns that we allow to permeate the future, the traumas that we might be too afraid or busy to address, will continue in our children's lives. The current state of the planet is the most obvious example of what can happen when previous generations blindly pass on unfinished psychic or energetic baggage. A tremendous opportunity has arisen for you to become an influencer of the future: your unique voice and history must be heard.

# Spiritual Fertility Essentials

Trauma can be passed down from the generations that came before us. While our ancestral line often works to support us, sometimes the trauma we inherit impacts our fertility. This chapter taught you how to identify inherited trauma by investigating the history of your family, as well as the timeline of your own conception, birth, and life. Paying special attention to cyclical events and anniversaries, as well as similarities in major life events such as miscarriage and death, provides a clear window into patterns that have yet to be healed within your family line.

As we identify and work through the energetic wounds from our family, we begin to heal the impact this trauma has had on our energy body and our endocrine system. This healing works inversely, as well, reaching back in time to the many generations that came before us. Identifying and clearing transgenerational trauma and trauma from our own birth also prepares the path for a healthier pregnancy by creating clearer boundaries between ourselves and our family lines. At this point, you should be able to begin identifying whether the energetic trauma you are carrying is your own or your ancestors'.

# Chapter 3

# Psychological and Energetic Blocks to Becoming Pregnant

While it is common to inherit some transgenerational trauma, injury in a person's current life can create an entirely different form of energetic blockage. Many people have deep and often-unspoken shame, blame, and guilt around unresolved traumas. Unfortunately, some come to the false conclusion that these blockages are why they are experiencing infertility, even though they have never been given tools to work through and release the trauma. And when they try to share this with doctors, spouses, and friends, they are often shut down and dismissed instead of empowered to trust their bodies and intuition. Spiritual fertility acknowledges these unseen factors and teaches you how to hold space and heal these invisible wounds.

As I started to write this chapter, I felt overwhelmed with a sense of responsibility to address everyone's experience with trauma fairly and compassionately. I have my own clinical experience and opinion as to which categories of trauma I believe impact the energetics of fertility the greatest; however, I also know that verbal, physical, and sexual trauma are experienced uniquely by individuals depending on their age, vulnerability, and when the trauma takes place in relation to developmental milestones.

I spent many days meditating, asking my guides to direct me to the common core of all traumatic events in each of our individual lives. I asked questions like: How do you take into account the fact that everyone's suffering is relative? How can we acknowledge that events that deeply injure one person are imperceptible to another person? As painful as trauma can be, might there be a greater purpose or a karmic role that it can play in the unfolding of our purpose here on Earth?

Days went by where I sat at my computer blankly, unable to write. One afternoon I took a break for my daughter's kindergarten parent/teacher conference. I walked over to the school classroom and sat down at the tiny kid-size table across from Cindy, my daughter's teacher. We spoke for some time about reading, math, and interpersonal skills—all fairly standard stuff—but toward the middle of the meeting, the energy shifted and Cindy's voice began to soften.

I've trained myself over the years to recognize moments like these as important messages from the universe. People in your life will often deliver the feedback you have been seeking if you simply hold the space and listen intently, as you would at a play, a concert, or a sermon. Cindy was about to convey wisdom about trauma as only a seasoned kindergarten teacher could: through a story.

"Imagine," Cindy said, "that you are sitting at this table and you see a shiny red apple resting at the edge that keeps rolling off and hitting the ground. Even though it keeps getting picked up and placed back on the table, you know that it's bruised inside because you have seen it fall. Now, imagine that someone new comes through the door and sees the same shiny red apple on the table but has absolutely no idea that it is injured inside. The same is true with how words and actions affect us," she continued. "Just because we look okay on the outside doesn't mean we are okay inside."

As Cindy was offering, injurious words can hurt us— and they begin very early in our social interaction with the world. Words are an extension of energy and emotion. As discussed in Chapter 2, children often express symptoms of trauma *for* the family—meaning that because children don't completely individuate until adolescence, it's difficult for them to filter what they hear and see in their homes and in the world. Thus, you can often see the undercurrents of what the home environment is like in a child's actions at school and with friends.

Among children, we tend to separate the bullied from the bully, but the truth is, they are two sides of the same trauma coin. That coin itself is like leftover change that has been passed down from a broken bill.

Many of the extensive and more violent traumas that occur later on in adolescence and through adulthood are an extension of the primary energetics of childhood. Children that show extreme sensitivity to the words of others, but who are never given tools to energetically and verbally protect themselves, are less likely to speak up in situations where they feel scared or injured. A loud and mean bully who is permitted to continue without intervention is more likely to inflict increasingly injurious degrees of trauma.

As you enter into conversations about becoming pregnant, wounds you experienced as a child and through adulthood can come to light. Many of these traumas might remain unspoken or even unconscious, but identifying and speaking of them now can be extremely healing, not only for your fertility but for your overall being.

Many of the topics I speak of in the remainder of this chapter will be relevant in one or more categories of trauma. Some parts of a story might resonate as true to you, while the other parts might seem inapplicable. Your fertility is a unique and elegant record of you that is not the same as anyone else's. Remember that your intuition is your greatest guide and no one, especially people in positions of authority, can tell you what is ultimately true for you unless it resonates as such.

### NAMING THE TRAUMAS THAT CONTRIBUTE TO INFERTILITY

While many traumas can impact humans, this section will focus on the traumas that tend to affect fertility. Namely, these are traumas that injure or break the fluid energetic connection between the mind, heart, ovaries, and uterus. Examples of traumas incurred in this lifetime are:

- Sexual assault
- Abortion/miscarriage/traumatic delivery
- Reproductive medicine
- Medical/pharmaceutical trauma

- Verbal abuse

- Psychological imbalance

- Shame around gender

- Environmental trauma and exposure

- Broken home

- Early exposure to pornography and graphic content

- Oppressive religious concepts

- Forced removal from home

- Loss of parent

Several traditional medical systems, such as Ayurveda and traditional Chinese medicine (TCM), have long acknowledged unseen pathways of connection between the seat of reproduction in the lower chakras and the house of the eternal spirit in the higher chakras. These pathways act much like electrical lines, smoothly delivering information, light, and power in response to the flick of a switch.

The connection between the emotions, mind, and reproductive center is significant. I use female sexuality as an example of this connection. For many women, if something feels off, if the heart feels injured, or if there is a great deal of stress, it is difficult to achieve orgasm. Likewise, for many women, having sex for the first time is hardly ideal—and rarely does it occur in an empowered, respectful, and healthy way. However, the means by which the experience is integrated greatly depends on your mental and emotional capacity to process and speak about the experience. This is also where a loving and supportive community and family can hold space for you and help to support you without blame, shame, or guilt.

For those who had no choice in deciding to have sex, who were pressured or forced to, the initial energetic imprint and initiation of the system that controls fertility is forever influenced by this initial contact and trauma. Unfortunately, the younger the age during which this imprinting occurs, the longer it can take to excavate and heal: it is, however, always capable of being healed.

One of the important windows that opens when you have difficulties getting pregnant is the ability to finally identify, name, and heal deep trauma. I highly recommend working with a skilled acupuncturist, therapist, or healer who is capable of acknowledging the role of trauma in the mind and body connection.

What we know of the endocrine system also supports the concept of connection between the mind, heart, and uterus. The pineal gland and hypothalamus, which act as master regulators, are located in the space behind the third eye and are in constant communication with the uterus and ovaries. While this connection is not as literal as the energy meridian that is drawn in an acupuncture diagram, it can be seen very clearly in the pathways that the hormones estrogen, progesterone, testosterone, and adrenaline take in the body. *Hormone* literally translates to "messenger" from Greek, giving it the extremely important task of courier and mediator between the outside world and the internal secret world of the reproductive system.

Nature is beyond intelligent. Above all else, as I work with individuals year after year, I have seen evidence of this elegant, sophisticated intelligence. The body has intuitively evolved to identify signals from the environment, including the emotional triggers of fear, shock, and danger, which can indicate an unsafe environment for a pregnant woman. Factors that are threatening for a mother and baby—including excessive stress, lack of nourishment, and exposure to the elements—are translated through the hormone cortisol to the endocrine system as an alarm bell to delay or block ovulation so pregnancy will not occur. In the best-case scenario, once the threat has passed, this temporary block should lift; however, sometimes it does not and the endocrine system continues to operate as if it were under attack. The more severe and prolonged the trauma, the longer it can take the blockage to lift and the system to reset.

## WHEN TRAUMAS ARE CAUSED BY THE MEDICAL SYSTEM

Many traumas that impact fertility are directly related to modern medicine. I often say that the infertility epidemic is the end result or unintended consequence of the sexual revolution. In 1968, when oral birth control became accessible to the general public, it was championed as an empowering tool for family planning and choice. And for many, it was. However, if we look at the underlying energetics of what oral birth control is directing the female body to do—that is, to halt ovulation and to thicken and reinforce otherwise soft and receptive membranes and fluids—we can imagine how, after decades of use, our biology would begin to adapt and incorporate this mediated relationship to fertility.

"The mind follows the body and the body follows the mind" is a quote widely used in holistic medicine to explain the influence that each system has on the other. This is especially true of the communicative hormonal system.

The lineage of fear and how we treat our young women around the time of menarche (when the menstrual cycle begins) is often the first incidence of microtrauma. A 39-year-old patient described her terror of becoming pregnant from a very young age, because her mother, who had been a teen mom, misled her into believing that having sex, regardless of where she was in her cycle, would lead to pregnancy. Instead of educating young women about the rhythm of their hormones and the innate wisdom of their biology, society often teaches us to be afraid and guarded about our sexuality and reproductive capacity.

Fear is the greatest cause of injury to the line of communication between the brain, heart, and uterus. We have not yet learned as a society that the only true way to prevent unfavorable and painful acts is through education and empowerment—not fear tactics, bullying, and peer pressure. Unsurprisingly, the patient who was taught to be terrified of sex was also put on oral birth control at 16 and stayed on it continuously until age 36, even though she did not become sexually active until age 21 and was only intermittently active afterward.

For her, the decision to have a child was complex, and although I sensed a sincere desire to become a mother (as well as the presence of a child's spirit), I also strongly felt that her indecisiveness was directly related to her relationship with her own mother and her early fears around reproduction. In this case, and many others, I have directly seen that oral birth control can reinforce psychological and energetic traumas to the reproductive system. A very important clinical question that reveals to what degree oral birth control might be reinforcing trauma is: How long does it take your body to start having a regulated period after coming off of birth control? The longer it takes, even and especially if you were placed on birth control to help regulate your cycle, the more likely it is that birth control was covering up or masking a more deeply rooted injury to your endocrine system. While I do not believe oral contraceptives create infertility, they can strongly reinforce the energetics that do.

Abortion is another topic that often comes to light when working with fertility. Over the years, I have heard so many women (when allowed a supported space) speak about their fear that the abortions they had in the past, regardless of whether their reasons were personal or medical, are contributing to their inability to conceive. Most doctors, because of lack of evidence, quickly rule out past abortions as a cause; typically, reproductive medical doctors are even glad to know that a woman's body was able to conceive naturally, even if the pregnancy was terminated. However, I support the intuition of my patients. If part of them "knows" that a previous abortion is contributing to infertility, then we incorporate this hunch into our sessions.

Just as oral birth control can reinforce energetics that contribute to infertility, abortion is a controversial trigger topic in society. Its history and controversy make it an obvious potential trauma for someone to experience. For many people, terminating a pregnancy feels shameful. In addition to the intense medical procedure—which is often navigated without the support of a partner or family—abortion often occurs during a traumatic time in a person's life, such as a breakup or unsupportive relationship, medical reasons, excessively busy or hectic period in a person's career, accidents influenced by substance abuse, sexual assault, and so on.

In a perfect world, I advise a woman choosing to undergo an abortion to take space and time around the procedure to heal with the support of a professional therapist or birth worker, such as a doula. Many doulas are now trained in supporting women both physically and psychologically through all procedures involving the uterus, such as hysterectomy, fibroid removal, miscarriage, and abortion. Having an experienced and compassionate shoulder to lean on can be instrumental to a healthy recovery.

The environment of trauma in which the abortion takes place does influence fertility, but it is not related to any moral, energetic, or karmic consequence. Many women have asked me over the years if the spirit of the child they terminated is still with them, potentially affecting their future fertility. I always inquire in return, "Do you think their spirit is lingering?" I believe and trust people's intuition, especially when it comes to their children. In many cases, there is no attachment from the spirits of past pregnancies, be they terminations or miscarriages, that impacts future fertility. However, if there is some attachment that a person feels, I recommend a ritual that I call the karmic archives, to release the energy and clear any remaining attachments (see sidebar page 60). Typically, what is influencing the future is the unfinished healing from the time around the abortion, which can always be revisited and healed.

Secrets, experiences, and beliefs that we each have, especially the ones that we are ashamed of and are afraid to admit, can lodge deep inside our spirit. Life will continue to present us with opportunities to heal these unfinished processes, including in the decision to become pregnant and carry that child from womb to first breath.

Lacey was a 32-year-old client who came to me utterly shut down and depressed after three failed embryo transfers. She was discouraged by the feeling of being broken, even though her doctors assured her that everything looked 100 percent normal in her lab tests and scans. Her husband and doctors were pushing her to continue with another round immediately, but luckily, she found me. We came up with a plan to help her find tools to return to IVF in a more autonomous way.

Reproductive medicine can be traumatic to experience, in and of itself. The high doses of hormones, ultrasounds, injections, and packed waiting rooms full of anxious and often upset people are not easy to remain unaffected by, especially when you are empathic. Lacey told me of her childhood growing up on a farm and described her early life as being extremely healthy. But in her young adulthood, a failed relationship resulted in an unwanted pregnancy that she chose to terminate without any support from friends or family. She shared that the desire to be a mother had been very strong for her since she was young, and that she felt she had betrayed her child by turning away. To her, the failure with IVF confirmed that she had done something that could not be forgiven—and that, in fact, she was now being punished for it.

We sat in deep meditation together and revisited the little girl on the farm, as well as the young woman alone in the doctor's office. We discovered the common thread between the two: music. I encouraged her to write a lullaby to her child, an exercise that I have given to many people over the years (see page 65). The power of song transcends the material world and can facilitate a direct connection to spirit. Lacey discovered that she was able to move past all her guilt with the comfort of knowing that she could still sing to her child's spirit. As she later shared with me, she recorded and listened to the melody on headphones during the next embryo transfer, which was successful.

## Exercise: *The Karmic Archives*

To clear the remnants of energetic attachments that might be lingering in your body and spirit, visit the karmic archives (sometimes known as the Akashic Records). Visualize a grand library in the sky. Imagine a place like the Library of Congress that is large enough to hold the history of human experience.

As you enter the magnificent front doors, you are given a pass to travel unsupervised anywhere you like in the "stacks." Your next step is to find the files containing details about the energy that is reluctant to release its attachment to you. Imagine each file to be a thought or a memory related to the energy that you are trying to clear. Keep following your train of thought, linking one memory to the next, all while continuing to visualize pulling these files out of the archives. When you feel like you have found all relevant information, imagine carrying your files toward the back of the library.

As you open the rear entrance, you will see a massive fire surrounded by four "head librarians." These librarians have the power to clear away any material that is no longer relevant to your healing path and your life's purpose. They are there to witness the removal of unneeded attachments and support you in cleaning house. Ask them to notarize your action as you throw the files that you collected into the fire, destroying them forever.

You can return back to the stacks as many times as you need if another thought, picture, or memory surfaces. With time, you will notice that there is nothing left to burn and that the chapter of your life that seemed impossible to get through has become nothing but a distant dream. The story will always influence your life, but you will never have a need for that book again.

## HEARTBREAK AND WOMB BREAK

Speaking about trauma can be difficult. As I mentioned, the body has amazing and complex fail-safe systems to conserve and protect an individual. And while many of our core systems as humans are similar, our unique and individual contributions can be more complex to disentangle. Some of this contribution is the result of the ancestral line in which you were born, as we mentioned in Chapter 2, but it also has a great deal to do with your spirit and the agreements that you have made for this lifetime (a topic we will cover in Chapter 9).

Post-traumatic stress disorder (PTSD) and its connection to fertility remains unexplored territory. Traumatic experiences, especially those that involve the womb, such as sex and childbirth, impact an individual forever. I call this womb break.

When I speak with people seeking an initial consultation, I can almost always identify those who have experienced womb break. Such was the case of 33-year-old Sarah, who called me from California. She immediately thanked me for my time, repeating on several occasions in the first minutes of the call that she didn't want to be a bother. I assured her she could never be. She spoke quickly, as though she had to fit as much information in as efficiently as possible, her voice strained and exhausted. Sarah went on to describe her story of secondary infertility, which occurs when a person experiences infertility after having had a successful prior pregnancy. Her story had much in common with others: getting pregnant easily the first time, and experiencing frustration with not being able to conceive again, after 12 months of trying. Her reproductive medical doctor diagnosed her with low ovarian reserve and recommended using a donor egg. Sarah was

61

confused and greatly distrustful of her body. She already had a two-year-old daughter, and her lifelong desire to have children close in age was quickly slipping away. She described feeling like she had a "gun to my head," with respect to how she should proceed.

"Sarah," I said, "slow down. I can hear that you have not been listened to by your doctors, and I can sense that you went through something extremely traumatic. We have all the time in the world, but first I want you to take a few deep breaths and tell me, without overthinking it, why you think you are not able to get pregnant?"

She began to cry. "How did you know that my daughter's birth was traumatic?"

I quietly held space as she continued: "I had to be put on antidepressants when my daughter was six months old. I'd never had a problem with mental health before her birth, but I had an emergency C-section; the anesthesia didn't work and I felt everything. It was terrifying, and I was so scared and unable to get over the experience. I've felt so guilty and ashamed for not being able to be okay. I really want my daughter to have a close sibling, but I can't go through childbirth again. I just can't do it."

For many rational minds, this type of PTSD could not possibly be the cause of infertility, but the powerful connection between the brain, heart, and uterus is truly under-recognized. I've worked with thousands of patients over the years and was trained to take medical histories by observing not only what patients report in words, but also how they look, sound, feel, and smell. My medical training activates when I hear a case like Sarah's, and I begin to look for underlying and prior diagnoses, as well as medical conditions that could have gone undiagnosed. However, even if there might have been an underlying condition, the kind of PTSD that Sarah experienced is enough to block fertility, and to disrupt hormone levels and radically reduce ovarian reserve. My initial intuition while speaking to Sarah was that the amount of trauma she had endured might prevent her from ever carrying a pregnancy, even with a donor egg, to term. Moreover, I felt a great deal of concern for the health of her family and young daughter, who had also been impacted by this experience. I knew that Sarah could recover and heal the trauma with time, but that the stress and physical demands of a second pregnancy could actually seriously endanger her mental and physical health.

I had already learned through the painful loss of a dear friend, Adrienne, that postpartum depression is the second leading cause of death, via suicide, in mothers of young children. I am also all too aware of how a mother who appears to be managing can be hiding a universe of pain and despair.

I responded, "Sarah, I'm not by any means suggesting that you will not be pregnant again, but what I do want to work on is imagining a possible reality where you don't have another biological child. I know that you will feel a lot of grief around this, but let's explore what the next year could look like if, right here and now, you stopped trying."

Silence on the phone.

"I thought you helped people like me, the hardest cases, to magically have babies," she said.

"I do," I replied, "and for you, this is where the magic begins."

Sarah, like so many women I work with, is a warrior, although she would never describe herself that way. The hardest and most difficult battles on Earth are fought in our own hearts and minds. Being honest with ourselves—honest to the very seed of the soul with which we came to Earth—sometimes feels impossible. When we experience only being loved when we meet certain milestones or conditions that others have for us (such as marriage, career, or the number of children we have), it can become harder and harder to express this self-knowledge.

Becoming a parent opens your heart in ways that you often did not know was possible. As the heart opens to love, the floodgates open and the places where it had been broken in the past often become more obvious. In this vulnerability and receptivity, self-reflection and inquiry can bear fruit. This is why so many people who have had children describe parenthood as an experience of continually having their hearts break open: through love, grief, and also expansion and self-realization.

The weight of trauma is undeniable. Trauma is not a simple emotion that allows one to quickly shrug it off and happily move on. Trauma has the power to stop a person's unfolding life in its tracks with a chilling slowness. This slowness is by design, granting an opportunity to create the time and space that are often needed to process experiences on the mental and physical level. Although technology and digital communication have not changed the amount of space and time necessary to process trauma, space and time themselves have become somewhat antithetical to modern life. Identifying trauma is as simple as asking yourself to take an honest inventory of the experience. How much time did you allow yourself to process the trauma? Who did you share it with, and were you totally honest about how the trauma impacted your life? Mending your heart is essential to preventing future trauma, but there is not a stopwatch measuring the speed at which you heal. Take your time, and know that you are supported by the universe.

## Exercise: *Compose a Lullaby*

Compose a lullaby for your unborn child. In this song, you are free to express all of your longing and love without any shame or fear. Start finding a melody through humming, building on it with words. Think of this lullaby as a letter you are directly addressing to your child. What prayer or mantra do you want your little one to hear? Sing the song either out loud or to yourself whenever you are feeling discouraged and in need of hope. Record it on your phone and listen to it when you need support and centering. If this truly feels like an impossible exercise, adopt a lullaby that has already been created and make it your own.

Remember that song transcends the atmosphere in which it is created and rises all the way to heaven. Your lullaby will soothe and comfort your child's spirit, as well as your own. It will also act as a beacon to help call your baby home.

## POST-TRAUMATIC GROWTH AND HEALING, AND HOW IT RELATES TO THE PLANET

Trauma impacts all of us differently. While some of us might have better coping mechanisms, we usually judge their efficacy by our ability to be successful and functional in society. This is not a terrible way to keep score, but it does beg the question as to if and how we as a global society actually want to heal our deepest wounds rather than simply operate as functional beings in the world.

I mention all of this because I have seen that there is no better place to witness the intersection between individual trauma and collective trauma than in fertility.

When the very sustainability of the Earth depends on its habitation by conscious and healthy humans, our unique paths through fertility directly impact the collective. One person's inability to conceive is reflective of a greater universal imbalance, and one person's healing within fertility radically impacts the future.

As a medical intuitive and a doctor, I have seen firsthand the interconnectedness of the health of the planet and the health of my patients. Events that impact the collective affect us all. The last two chapters have dwelled on the impact of trauma on each of us. I champion the individual, and I believe that one of the most profound ways of impacting the world is to follow our own individual paths of healing and purpose with integrity. As you identify potential traumas and how you may or may not have processed those wounds energetically and psychologically, hold space for yourself and recognize that your traumas are also the world's traumas. This by no means minimizes your experience; on the contrary, it can empower you to see the bigger picture that has been at play on the planet. As you create a new dream for your own life and family, you can include a new potential path for all those who share the Earth with you, as well.

I began this book with the intention of teaching you how to become your own intuitive healer and to describe clear methods for connecting with the spirit of your child while still living in the modern, rational world. There are many opportunities to mend decades-old hurt through your individual healing. While fertility is one of the greatest ways to do this, you can also heal by focusing on your own physical, mental, and spiritual health.

Nothing that we experience is without purpose. Every great teacher I have studied reiterates that all events we observe, especially the hardest and darkest ones, are opportunities for growth. Our greatest injuries and losses occur to keep us on our spiritual path, and when we don't experience pain and stress, we simply do not grow. But because we are all connected intimately, the myth that somehow your suffering is your own fault and responsibility is plainly wrong. Evolutionary biology teaches us that a unique brilliance that can manifest in a successful person might present in that person's sibling as mental illness and an inability to be functional in the world. In other words, each of us is on a unique path that is determined by a number of factors, environmental and spiritual.

You don't have to address the more difficult memories from your past in order to become pregnant and have a healthy child; in fact, when you look around it becomes clear that most blindly jump into pregnancy and child-raising. Over the years, many people have asked me why, after taking the decision to become a parent extremely seriously and only heading into the agreement of parenthood after years of psychological and physical healing, others who seemingly have not done this type of conscious conception work tend to get pregnant more easily and without delay. I always respond with an old Texas saying: "You can't cross the bridge until you get to the river." Ultimately, conceiving a child, no matter how much work we have put into our healing and our health, is an issue of cosmic timing, a topic we will explore in depth later. Letting go and trusting in this timing is one of the very first lessons of parenthood: a lesson that we are more prepared to learn if we have reflected and healed the wounds of a lifetime.

## Spiritual Fertility Essentials

When we start to enter the conversation about becoming a parent, our past wounds and traumas can resurface. And while everyone experiences trauma, for some of us, trauma takes time to heal. The experience of getting pregnant and having a child presents us with a passageway into conscious and unconscious trauma that we might be carrying, and it also shows us the path to healing.

In this chapter, you learned how to identify trauma that might be buried in blame, shame, and guilt—and how to shed a healing and nonjudgmental light onto its purpose in your life's path. We explored the connection between the emotions, mind, and reproductive center. You learned that becoming your own advocate is essential to navigating fertility and motherhood. When you reconnect to your spirit and your intuition, you tap into a reservoir of energy and power that is meant to protect you and guide your way. Trauma need not be seen as something negative or shameful in your life story, but rather, it can be a testament to your strength of spirit and your ability to autonomously heal the wounds of the past.

# Chapter 4

# The Impact of Our Most Intimate Relationships on Our Fertility

People are often surprised that when I begin to discuss the importance of healing relationships in fertility, I usually speak about relationships other than a person's marriage or primary romantic partnership. The three fundamental relationships that I address, in order of importance, are:

- Your relationship/lack of relationship to God/ the universe

- Your relationship/lack of relationship to your parents (particularly your mother)

- Your relationship/lack of relationship to your partner

Becoming comfortable with all facets of intimacy and vulnerability (not just our relationship with our primary partner) is a fundamental building block of letting go of the need to control, which is so important in the fertility process. Intimacy is a reflection of our ability to connect to a deep internal space; from this space, we can recognize what feels familiar in the world—and once we identify it, we can begin to draw it in through the most powerful universal law: love.

Our very first relationship is to the infinite, and this relationship plays a major role in fertility. From our primary relationship with ourself, we build our universe, which includes the people, place, and time we are born into. The worldly relationships that have a major impact on our desire to have a child reflect something about our own spiritual path. As you decide to enter into the new relationship of parenthood, remember that what you and your future children have in common is that you are both born from spirit and will both return to spirit. For many people, the concept of an eternal soul, or a soul that can reincarnate, is uncomfortable because it is not tangible or confirmed by science. An important step in working with energy, especially the energy of helping draw in your child's spirit, is taking the risk in believing that an eternal soul does, indeed, exist. As with all that I suggest in my teachings of spiritual fertility, I am not asking you to be a true believer. It is not necessary for you to unquestioningly follow any of what I suggest. Indeed, the point of spiritual fertility practices is to ultimately strengthen your connection to intuition to such an extent that you only accept advice when it resonates as true with your mind, heart, and spirit. For some of you who already have a spiritual practice that acknowledges the before- and afterlife, the notion that your child's spirit exists is not a particularly difficult one to digest. But for others, including many I have worked with over the years, this concept is hard.

Perhaps you can observe this disconnect in your own life. Maybe in your partnership, you have a spiritual way of approaching the world while your partner is more rational or cynical—or vice versa. We are often karmically attracted to people who can trigger our unresolved issues. As the poet Rumi writes, "Things are revealed by their opposite."

There is no better opportunity to resolve our issues, especially about relationships, than in the decision to consciously create. Many of our relationships that feel antagonistic or that challenge us to process unacknowledged trauma can benefit from the reminder that our most important and fundamental relationship is the one we have to the Divine. Acknowledging this primary connection is a diplomatic gesture to the infinite, a simple action that demonstrates your readiness to listen and evolve. We can approach all conversations and difficulties we have with ourselves, our partners, and the spirits of our future children in the same way. Indeed, demonstrating respect and compassionate listening can heavily influence the outcome of every conversation we have.

## YOUR RELATIONSHIP TO THE DIVINE

Our first relationship as individual human beings existed before we were born. This bond encompassed the space, time, and territory of all that which came before our first breath. All of your relationships with others begin with your relationship to the Divine. This primary relationship sets the stage for all other subsequent relationships. It's easy to get more complicated than this, critiquing and blaming the other people in our lives—even those with whom you share the greatest intimacy—for all the possible reasons that you have not found happiness, are not getting pregnant, or why so many things in the world can go wrong.

The greatest ally you have in life is your own spirit and its relationship to the universe, but it's easy to lose sight of this in the midst of fertility issues. For many of my clients, the first time they truly experience not getting what they want, when they want it, is when they don't become pregnant within a certain period of time. It's hard to feel the call to motherhood—and to already have so many important components of building a family established (a stable partner, economic security, comfortable home, good career, and so on)—and to not have it happen.

Most people's first reaction to not getting pregnant is anger. This is usually expressed against their partner and the unfairness of other people easily conceiving, even though they are seemingly not as prepared to be parents. Anger can generate change, and in this respect I think it is a powerful force in working within fertility.

I would be remiss if I didn't mention the underlying energetics of the male/female relationship when it comes to anger around sexuality and fertility. The patriarchal structure that has dominated Western culture has not left much room for feminine expression, and much of the feminist response to past oppression has been fueled by anger, which is a powerful changemaker. However, the slippery slope of blaming and projecting the history of inequality between men and women onto your present fertility leads to a dead end. I never counsel my clients to mitigate their anger toward their partners, their boss, or global politics. But I do ask them to step back and instead catalyze their anger as a healing force in developing a new intimacy with their own spirit.

Anger, while an undeniable driver of change, can also stagger your personal development and hinder intimacy with your partner, family, and the world. I myself have felt the impacts of the anger that originated in the experiences I had growing up as a preacher's kid in a religion that didn't see women as equal. I understood the teachings of the Bible to be about equality, fairness, and spiritual liberation. The hypocrisy of people using these core values for their own gain threw me into rebellion and spiritual crisis.

When I became an adult, many unresolved feelings of my childhood often played out in my relationships, particularly anger. Through deep analysis, I discovered that the epicenter of my anger was not my partner or my parents, but my relationship with the Divine. The initial mystical experiences I'd had, of feeling spirit in all things, was ripped out from under me by people, politics, school, and the sadness of the world. Anger, while my greatest defense against all of this, was merely a cover for the sadness and distrust I felt and the underlying belief that I was actually not supported by the universe.

I was ultimately angry at God.

## TRANSFORMING ANGER INTO SELF-CARE

Years later, when I was in the third row of a Tori Amos concert in New York City, she said something between songs that touched me deeply. The album for which she was touring contained songs about environmental devastation and our lack of stewardship of the Earth, but as she spoke, she described how she turned her anger into action through song—and how she was inspired to do this for her daughter: "I had to create another story, another potential path for the future, one of hope."

This resonates for me and many of my clients. Our children follow the generalized paths that we carve, and while anger has been valuable and can dynamically enact change, it is what we decide to do with this anger that determines our path.

Anger tends to be the first emotion that percolates to the surface in relationships when we are not getting our essential needs meet. The consciousness that you develop with yourself creates a strong foundation for your conception and pregnancy, and also influences the development and consciousness of your child.

People speak of self-care frequently these days, but I see self-care as a timeless personal practice for carving out the space and solitude necessary for listening to your spirit. It creates the internal dialogue to dream up something better for your life and for the Earth. Without this internal dialogue and the space to listen, intimacy with others is close to impossible. None of this can be done if your reservoir is running low or is dangerously depleted. How can you give freely of love and compassion if you have not first experienced it in your own heart? The practice of self-care is about creating a consistent monitoring system. The tools that you discover become a method for calibrating your energetic scales. Observing when the scales tip from one side to another often gives you the insight to determine what is out of alignment in your life.

Just because you practice consistent self-care, and see imbalance as it happens, doesn't necessarily mean you will prevent depletion. As I wrote this section, I noticed that I let my phone run out of energy, although I was expecting an important call. My normal routines and practices I need to keep me anchored sometimes get thrown out the window, especially when I am busy. It is important to acknowledge that free will is always at play. Even when we choose not to care for ourselves, or decide to place others' needs before our own, we are always demonstrating this free will.

## Exercise: *Finding Your Pillars*

This is a tool that I developed for myself after the birth of my daughter. I was overwhelmed with responsibility and unable to prioritize my own care. I needed a practice that was simple and easy to remember. I consulted a tarot deck and pulled the High Priestess card. It reminded me that ancient temples and churches followed a clear and methodical orientation. They were often built to model the heavens and arranged in accord with the directions. These foundations created the space for higher-level connection to self and the spirit.

Sacred spaces are meant to inspire a life that mirrors humanity as a reflection of the holy. I was yearning for inspiration and clarity as to how to remain balanced and found that it was as simple as cleaning my house.

Determine the pillars of what you absolutely need in order to support the structure of your spirit. I suggest finding at least four that you can practice daily. To help determine what your pillars are, think back to the times of your life when you were happiest and most in alignment with your spirit. Remember the things you were doing, the food you were eating, the places where and people with whom you were spending time. Identify your pillars and write them down. Do not compromise on integrating these pillars into your life. I have found that I can go a few days without one or two, but after that, I begin to see cracks in my foundation and my temple feels compromised.

I have a personal practice I call Finding Your Pillars (see sidebar on page 75), that is an extremely helpful form of self-care. I developed it in the first year of my daughter's life, when I found myself prioritizing everyone in my life before myself. Practicing essential love and conscious care for yourself before you get pregnant will create a foundation to carry this practice through pregnancy and parenthood.

## YOUR RELATIONSHIP TO YOUR PARENTS

"What is your relationship like with your mother?" is a question I ask my patients frequently, and the range and complexity of answers is very telling. We follow the energetics of our parents, and the example they set heavily influences our belief systems around what is possible for our own lives. But even more specifically, the transition in consciousness that occurs when you become a parent opens up deep memories from your earliest time on the planet and often triggers new ways of relating to your parents.

Many people find themselves capable of reaching a new level of compassion for their parents once they become parents themselves. The difficulty of navigating parenthood, combined with the reality of living in a world that does not support women and families, is a painful reality that can only truly be understood once experienced. Our greatest capacity for compassion is often rooted in shared life events. This is one reason that strong, long-lasting bonds develop with the tribe that supports you through infertility, pregnancy, and the raising of young children.

While some experience this compassion, for others entering into parenthood is an entirely different experience, one of clearer boundaries and, sometimes, the dissolution of relationships. Often, unresolved issues within our relationships only come to light when we look deeply into the root of our symptoms. If we don't heal these deeper injuries, we often unconsciously repeat the trauma, typically in the form of allowing relationships into our lives that keep us frozen and unable to evolve.

Brigitte called me one late summer day, looking for help. She had already been trying to get pregnant for six months but broke into tears halfway through the conversation, insisting that something felt off. She, like many others, was hesitant because she and her husband were uncertain about the extent to which they were prepared to use Western reproductive medicine, especially lab work.

I sensed from the start that Brigitte had unresolved trauma from a previous terminated pregnancy. Our first call together confirmed that she had experienced a termination at a young age, and that she had been susceptible to an abusive spiritual community—in particular, an older man who took advantage of her and impregnated her. Brigitte's spirit was fierce as a result of surviving abuse. She was the type of friend and partner who would fight to the death for you. But when it came to fighting for her own needs, both emotionally and physically, she was still extremely critical of her own perceived weaknesses.

Through the tools explored in Chapters 2 and 3, we worked to clear the leftover energetic connections from her early 20s. Just as we turned this corner, a huge wave of blocked and unresolved emotion flooded Brigitte's energetic field. It became clear in my intuitive vision that the spirit of her daughter, which I had felt connected to since our very first call, was ready to be born but did not feel welcomed. So I opened our next session by asking, "Why do you not want to have a girl?"

Brigitte was quiet for a bit but then said, "I had a dream a few days ago about my daughter, and I'm terrified because I know that she wants to be my child."

"What is terrifying about it?" I inquired.

"I was a terrible daughter," she explained, "and my mom told me all throughout my childhood that she hoped that I would have a daughter who was just as bad as I was so that I would suffer like she did."

"Aha," I responded. "This is it, Brigitte, the last piece of the puzzle."

For Brigitte, like many others, the hurt of a difficult childhood in a broken home—as well as the weight of being energetically sensitive without being given the tools, unconditional love, and encouragement necessary to learn how to channel and express this sensitivity—resulted in childhood behavior "problems." Her mother was not a bad mother, but was overworked, under-supported, and unable to supply Brigitte with the tools she needed. So she did what many parents do: lash out in anger and frustration.

Although Brigitte understood on some level that her mother's attitude was not truly about her, she had still taken her words to heart. A powerful practice known as re-parenting (see sidebar on page 79) ultimately led to a breakthrough moment for Brigitte. Through this exercise she became capable of stepping into the moments of her childhood through the eyes of her higher self, thus rewriting the narrative that her mother had imprinted on her. Together we reenacted the scenes from her childhood, changing the conversation to be supportive and loving instead of angry and judgmental. By the end, while she felt a new level of compassion for her mother, Brigitte also understood the ways in which her mother had failed to be a good parent for her when she needed it most. She was able to heal this lack of unconditional love by remembering that even at that time in her life, she was being held, loved, and watched over by God.

Re-parenting allows us to revisit scenes from our childhood and unpack the moments when our parents failed us. Allowing your present-day self to re-parent your inner child with love, respect, and patience heals deep wounds of shame and negative beliefs about yourself. It is an integral step to healing, especially when you become a parent. During her next cycle, Brigitte conceived a baby girl. She also inadvertently healed her relationship with her mother and was able to allow her back into her life with clear communication and newly set boundaries.

## Exercise: *Re-parenting*

Picture yourself as a child. Now imagine your present self as the parent of this younger self. Make an inventory of what has changed between your younger self and your older self. Visualize the moments when you were most hurt by the actions of your parents. How did they pass down judgment and anger instead of the love and patience that you needed? Can you determine the beliefs about yourself that you developed around that time? Was there a moment in childhood where things shifted for you significantly? For example, perhaps a move, change of school, or conflict in your family caused you to act out.

The practice of re-parenting enables you to return to this moment and allow a greater force to step in where your parents failed to be your advocate. Observe how your inner child feels when you experience unconditional love and support. When you are feeling self-critical and find yourself in a loop of negative beliefs, step in to be an advocate for yourself. Show yourself the unconditional love that you show others.

## SEX AND YOUR INTIMATE RELATIONSHIP

Most learned strategies designed to power through difficulty or perform better to achieve a goal simply do not work when it comes to infertility. Infertility is often the first experience people have of their learned strategies for success simply not working. This is one reason infertility can offer a valuable opportunity for a couple to closely examine their relationship priorities and overall quality of life.

We tend to idealize romantic relationships, and we project a lot of societally imposed expectations onto them. Western culture is centered around setting and reaching goals—and our entire economy supports this structure. We are taught the correct order of events should take place in life, beginning with graduating from school, finding a career and a partner, getting married, and then starting a family. If this structure breaks down, it can create a crisis. A healing opportunity that is rooted in suffering can change the direction of your life.

In Hinduism, the goddess Kali is known as the deity of destruction and death. It is Kali's job to keep you on your spiritual path through often-painful life events, such as the loss of a job, illness, and infertility. The deep lessons we learn when faced with these life challenges, and the opportunity we are given to deepen our relationship with ourself and our partner, are some of Kali's gifts. That is not to say that these experiences will magically stop sucking, or even that they will become easier with perspective. During such times, we will be prompted to dig deep—but through them, we will also grow and strengthen the most.

Sometimes, infertility is the symptom of a strained intimate relationship; other times, infertility is what creates the strain. A common effect of infertility is a sexless marriage or partnership. People often refer back to times before they began trying to become pregnant as "better" and "more fulfilling," emotionally and sexually. The pain that both members of a couple experience when pregnancy is not occurring can reinforce negative patterns within the relationship. One person can easily project their sadness and frustration onto the other, instead of sharing their internal emotional state.

Our sex life can offer us a lot of information about how we are relating to our partner, and can give us a tally of how much focused, undistracted time we are sharing with our loved one. Unfortunately, the ideal of having children can be treated as just another goal to obtain and tick off the list; this creates a split in our understanding that having children is related to being intimate with your partner. It is important to keep sex and intimacy fun and lighthearted, especially as people are trying to conceive. Partnership and marriage need to be prioritized *above* pregnancy, and love should always be emphasized as a powerful healing force. After all, the spirits of our children looking down upon us are attracted to loving partnerships and clear desire between two people.

However, for many, sex is layered with discomfort, trauma, broken trust, and unconscious issues in our intimate relationship. Mindy was referred by a colleague and was committed to getting to the bottom of why she was not getting pregnant. She took a long train ride into New York City to meet with me in person weekly for many months and never missed or rescheduled a session. Mindy was committed to healing on every level: physical, mental, and spiritual. On a physical level, her cycles were regular, and she had clear bifurcated follicular and luteal phases and positive ovulation tests. She had been married for five years and described her marriage as good; however, she and her spouse seemed to be in different places with respect to starting a family.

During the course of our work, I sensed a strong blockage in her energetic field that seemed to stem from her husband. She shared with me that he was very resistant to having a semen analysis and insisted that he was okay. After a period of working to improve her connection to her intuition, she decided to ask him again to get lab work done. At this time, he admitted that he had no interest in having children and that he was, in fact, having an affair and wanted a divorce. This was of course devastating for my client, but it confirmed what her intuition had been telling her all along.

They divorced quickly, and she moved forward with her life, unsure as to how and when she would have children. About a year later, she called me to say that she was five months pregnant and in love with an old friend. She described the work that we did together as imperative for the next step of her life and expressed gratitude for finding the path to connect to her spirit. She now has three children.

A resistant partner is not necessarily the wrong partner. The work of parenthood requires all hands to be on deck. Sometimes, one person is ready to have a family before the other, and this can cause discord, insecurity, and a lack of trust. Finding a way to communicate during this period is essential. I have witnessed that if couples speak about their hesitation and fears around parenthood prior to getting pregnant, this produces far better and faster outcomes once the timing is correct. The same applies to maintaining our connection and intimacy with a partner and prioritizing this bond when we are trying to conceive, be it through natural conception, assisted reproductive medicine, or the use of surrogacy.

The tendency to over-rationalize and explain through "science" how conception takes place de-emphasizes the power of love and romance. The spirit of your child knows how to identify and navigate a path to you via the emotion of love. Remember that to the spirit world, the laws and rules of humankind mean very little. We often over-complicate things with interpretation instead of allowing the energy to speak for itself.

Close your eyes for a moment and say these two statements aloud. First: "We have so much love between us that we have extra to share, and we want to share this love with you." Next say, "We really want you and are going to do everything the doctor and science say we need to do to conceive you." Which one feels more attractive, positive, and inclusive?

You can never go wrong with romance when it comes to connecting to your child's spirit. They love it and far prefer it to Excel spreadsheets, apps, and calendar alarms! Trust that the person you are with has been put into your life for the most extraordinary of purposes, which might be beyond your understanding—and allow this relationship to be a touchstone built on trust and love, regardless if you choose to have children or not.

Later in the book, we will dive into spirit contracts and how and why children's spirits are tied to specific parents. I want to state very clearly here that if your intuition is repeating over and over again that the reason you are not getting pregnant is that you are not meant to have a child with the particular partner you are with, then you need to listen to this voice. We live in a time of possibility and potential, and there are more ways than ever to pursue pregnancy. Whatever you might think, you do not have to stay with a partner who doesn't love you or who injures your spirit just because you are being loudly called to have a baby.

## CO-CREATING AND MANIFESTING YOUR
## RELATIONSHIP TO HUMANITY

Each of our communities provides a powerful source of herd immunity, encouragement, and support. These communities and relationships are all examples of what we have individually manifested and chosen. Each represents how well we are communicating our emotional, physical, and spiritual needs.

The experience of becoming a parent is transformational. It changes you and makes you question things you never did before . . . and this can create a strain in relationships where you are expected to remain the same. Because of this, relationships, especially the oldest and most relied on, are often tested.

I have found that becoming a mother pushed me to speak up and ask for what I needed, not just from my partner and family, but from the universe itself. After our daughter, Anna Libertine, was born, a friend asked me what I thought had changed the most.

"I can't explain it," I said, "but her birth educated my bones."

What I realize now is that the experience of pregnancy and birth awakened in me the knowledge of the most fundamental and foundational connections each human being has to every other human being and the Earth. When we remember that we are all created equal and that our relationships are here to help us celebrate and connect with each other, nothing is impossible. All of this begins with the acknowledgment that you and your connection to spirit are of utmost importance. Any partner, doctor, or family member who makes you feel like you are not important is simply someone to be removed from the phone book of your life. Asking for what you need, including support, is essential to your fertility. You are bringing to Earth more than just your own child; you are bringing in a fellow sister and brother to us all.

We have a choice in the types of relationships we allow in our lives. Sometimes fertility can provide us with an opportunity to shift the way we relate and with whom we choose to collaborate and create. Trusting your intuition is essential when evaluating the energies of others whom you allow into the sacred space of conception and pregnancy. This can be an energetically vulnerable time, and you might find that some of your relationships feel more unsupportive and draining than they did before. Your energy level is your guide. Allow space to be created for those who can show you unconditional love, and try to identify the relationships that are toxic and possibly working against you. You might not have to completely end those relationships; just identifying them will allow you to choose to what extent you want them in your life and the life of your child.

At times when I'm feeling exhausted and I've put my self-care on the back burner for too long, I'll remember the voice of my daughter saying to me, "Even if we are not together, we are always together."

I instantly know that she is correct—and I feel supported and loved. The types of relationships that we nurture for ourselves set the standard for the types of relationships our children nourish and facilitate in their lives. Simply remember that you have the power to manifest what you need, especially with respect to the relationships in your life. And is there any better example of the power of manifestation than that of conceiving a human being from spirit into flesh?

## Spiritual Fertility Essentials

Before we can consistently love others, our own reservoir must be full. It doesn't have to stay full all the time, but learning to notice when levels are dangerously low is essential for your spiritual well-being. In this chapter, we learned that everything starts with spirit. The fundamental relationship that exists between you and the numinous will influence all subsequent relationships in your lifetime.

Your connection to spirit and the universe is the most important relationship in your life. Repairing this relationship will heal all other relationships, including those with your family, partner, and children (born and unborn). You need not return to a spiritual or religious practice that you once lived by in order to renew this primary relationship, nor do you have to become a true believer in a new system; you simply need to have a practice to listen and connect to your intuition.

When we make time for ourselves, especially as mothers, we steer the ship for our entire family and karmic circle. In this space, you can alchemize anger into compassion and self-knowledge, but you must first find what it is that fills your own heart before you share your heart with others.

# Chapter 5

# Transforming Limiting Beliefs

Much of our modern society and culture is based on rational thought and empirical evidence, which can sometimes limit our capacity to understand factors outside of our mental comprehension. I have witnessed the powerful connection between people's belief systems and their health—and how their beliefs can either empower them and transform their lives, or do just the opposite. In many ways, this is the principle that drew me to practice holistic medicine instead of allopathic medicine.

Many times in my childhood, I was puzzled by the way people who held strong religious beliefs and exercised a faith-based life interacted with illness and disease. Frequently, it felt like there was a split between the spirit and the body, especially with respect to sexuality. I was curious as to how faith and spirituality interacted with science and rationalism. I was especially intrigued by what philosophy has termed the mind/body problem. Most of what we have been raised on in Western culture is the result of Cartesian dualism, which states that the mind and the body are two separate structures—a nice concept in theory but one that, in practice, seems unrealistic, especially in medicine.

The terrible asthma I experienced in my childhood and adolescence put me on my path as an energy healer and intuitive doctor. I often tell patients my story as an example of how our symptoms, or any illness, can help us along our spiritual and life journey. I graduated from high school early and went on to study philosophy and ethics in college at 16. I was thrilled to sit in classes that explored the history of ideas, knowledge, and spirituality. I was in the library researching the recent news of the completion of the Human Genome Project when I intuited that I needed to study medicine to understand how mind, body, and spirit all come together. Hence, I began taking all the premed requirements. During this time, I was still suffering from weak respiratory function and asthma, and a dear friend suggested I go to his traditional Chinese medicine (TCM) doctor. I was intrigued. This was a few decades ago, and acupuncture and Chinese medicine were nowhere near as well known then as they are today. I booked an appointment with Dr. Tina Baumgartner and showed up ten minutes late for a meeting that would change my life. I explained to her my history and everything I had done to treat my illness from a Western medicine standpoint, such as allergy shots, home nebulizers, and preventative steroid treatments. She listened and kindly nodded as I spoke.

"I'm not sure how you can help," I said at the end of my skeptical spiel.

She paused, took a deep breath, reached out, and warmly touched my hand before saying, "Julie, do you believe that you can heal your asthma?"

I have always been oddly tough, an attribute that many who are descendants of frontier people, settlers, and immigrants also share, but I found myself broken open by this question and the energy of this healer.

"No, I don't," I replied with tears streaming down my face. "But I want to."

"Then I can help you," she said.

Week after week, the "truth" that I had been told and that I believed about my body and health began to shift. I no longer felt that someone outside of me could take away my long-term illness. Ultimately, it was something that I had to tackle and heal myself. I discovered that there is a connection between emotions and our health, and that the more sensitive you are, the more sensitive the medicine you need. My limiting belief that I would always have asthma, which was supported by the opinions of Western allopathic doctors and my family, was a significant hurdle to jump. Leaving behind science and popular belief was terrifying. I mostly did it, like so many others who have explored alternative medicine, out of necessity. I just could not go on living an entire lifetime not being able to breathe.

I still look back in awe at the bravery of my younger self who when told "There is no cure for your asthma" stood up, left the doctor's office, and went out into the world to find one herself.

Every person I have treated shares this sovereignty in common. Each soul has followed the internal voice that says, "There must be something else I can do." There is beauty in looking deeply into the structure of what we have been taught to believe is true; we must question whether it really needs to be that way. Often, the answers we find are the very essence of what we need to heal. I needed to find a way to be given permission and to follow an unconventional path this lifetime, and the asthma I healed was my catalyst and my greatest teacher.

### INTUITION: A GATEWAY FOR HEALING AND RELEASING UNCONSCIOUS BELIEFS

In fertility, the same internal voice arises in many of my patients. Patients share with me that they don't believe they cannot conceive just because they are past what is considered the peak age of fertility. They often come to the conclusion that the diagnosis they have been given doesn't have to impact their fertility, and the stories of infertility that their friends and family have told them are not going to be their own stories.

No one out there knows more about life than you. "Experts" are passionate about what they do and teach—but none of their study, practice, or hard work can compete with your intuitive knowing. I'm sharing this with you, dear reader, because I want this book to provide you with permission for connecting and trusting in the intuition of your mind, body, and spirit as it pertains to connecting to the spirit of your child. What so many others call "miracles," I do not. While there is magic in the connection you have with your future child, the spiritual science that I have helped people navigate is rooted in real practices that all begin with one common seed: questioning a belief system that you or society holds as true.

The obviousness of our limiting beliefs tends to be available to us with just a little bit of self-exploration.

The deeper ones—the thoughts and feelings that are covered over by shame, blame, and guilt—are not as easy to uncover. I can psychically pinpoint and put a voice to these for many of my clients, but I feel that when I instead offer the correct prompts for them to speak it for themselves, it can be far more transformational. As a side note, this tends to be my perspective on using my intuitive channels in general. I prefer to empower people to connect with their own unique intuition, and I act as an advocate to remind them of that intuition when they are questioned by others or by their limiting belief systems. While there are profoundly compassionate and highly spiritual doctors in the realm of reproductive medicine, the default attitude, unfortunately, is the mind and body split that I talked about at the beginning of the chapter.

In addition, women's health concerns and perspectives in general still go unlistened to, and worse, judged by many doctors in both Western and alternative medicine as hysterical or fabricated. The best of the psychics I have learned from do not simply replicate the broken systems of Earth. They do not pride themselves on having access to a truth that you don't; rather, they inspire you to recall that you are a powerful channel yourself and help you to remember how to live in that empowered state.

It is just as important when looking at limiting unconscious beliefs to evaluate belief systems that we participate in with choice and consciousness. I work with people from all religious and spiritual backgrounds. Many who practice conventional religion are at first hesitant to work with energy medicine and intuitive forces. They often inquire in our initial contact about to what or whom I attribute my intuition and power. Belief systems that are rooted in monotheism are usually tentative when it comes to participating with people with practices outside of their belief systems.

Given my background as a Baptist preacher's daughter, I understand. It might be surprising for you to learn that, as supportive and loving as my parents are, there are still times when, no matter how successful I am at helping women connect with the spirits of their children, they are critical and fearful of my work. But the unconscious pattern that made me hesitant to share the gifts that I believe God gave me was broken the moment I helped a couple who had long experienced infertility to conceive and birth a healthy child through only the power of energy medicine. My journey is not about limiting who, how, and why a person can have a child; my job is to remind people that regardless of their religious or spiritual beliefs, or lack thereof, the only voice they truly need to hear and fight to protect is that of their unborn child. As far as I can tell, all the angels in the sky agree—and as it is above, so it is below. If you come from a traditional religious background, you do not need to fear or avoid your intuition. Rather, reframe your relationship to intuition and consider it a channel to help you hear God within, instead of a force that is separate from and outside of your belief system.

## THE LAW OF ATTRACTION AND COMMON PATTERNS OF LIMITING BELIEFS

The impact of our limiting beliefs on our fertility often begins with grave injury to our spirit. We usually set up parameters of what we believe can and cannot occur before we even start. Sometimes this information is available to us, and sometimes it is not. Remember Brigitte, who worked so hard to uncover the unconscious information that was blocking her from getting pregnant? The deep-seated belief, perpetuated by her mother, left Brigitte believing that if she were to have a daughter, the child would be poorly behaved and extremely hard to raise. This belief literally blocked Brigitte from conceiving.

Much of our modern society and culture is based on rational thought, which can sometimes limit our capacity to understand factors outside of our mental comprehension. I hesitate to list common limiting beliefs; anything that resides on the level of the unconscious fails to be well described in words. But I have observed specific themes within my practice.

Before we advance too far in helping you identify your own limiting beliefs about having children, I'd like to ask you the set of questions that I often begin with when helping my clients transform blockages. I've found that the answers to these questions are very telling as to where and why each client might be operating in a negative and limiting belief pattern. Take your time with each, and journal the answers as they come to you:

- What is the emotion that you are looking to feel when you imagine having a child?

- What will change in your life when you have a child?

- What will change in your relationships?

- Do you imagine feeling more complete, fulfilled, and happy once you have conceived? How so?

The answers to each of these questions are your first step in identifying the very thing you are looking for from the external world. Once you know that, you can begin to attract it into your life by finding a way to give it to yourself now, not later. As you recall from Chapter 4, the essential relationship you have is to your spirit. If we begin to look for emotional fulfillment or support from our children before they are ever born, we are setting ourselves up for disappointment. And, we are being unfair and demanding to the person whom we have yet to meet.

Baby spirits are brilliant. They have a sort of cosmic wisdom that reads energy and timing far better than we do here on Earth. I have noticed that certain souls, especially the ones who need extra support during this lifetime, wait for unconditional love. This requires each of us to be brutally honest with our real motives for having children.

Tibetan Buddhism, with its rich history of decoding the process of death and rebirth, describes several factors that must be present in order for conception to occur. One of these is that the unembodied spirit must sense purpose in being born to a couple. This purpose often is an extension of the work, or karma, of what this soul is seeking to complete in a lifetime. If a lack of this purpose is missing in a couple's life, I recommend that they return to acts of unconditional love and service to others in what I call the Mission of Kindness exercise (see sidebar on page 95). These acts open the heart and serve as a type of antidote to a self-centered and materialistic world. I had a lovely client once tell me that she knew that when she became a mother, she would be able to quit the corporate job she hated and finally do what she wanted to with her life: nurture and care for others. I explained that although it was beautiful that she felt so called to motherhood, unless she found a way now, before pregnancy, to practice this gift of nurturing, she would discover disappointment and depression after childbirth rather than the fulfillment she expected.

## Exercise: *Mission of Kindness*

Acts of service to others might seem like a strange fertility treatment, but I have found them to be an incredibly powerful healing tool. It is easy for any of us to get caught up in materialism and lose sight of what is essential about being alive. Sometimes returning to simple actions of kindness to help out a neighbor, a friend, or a family in need is powerful medicine for our own healing.

If you find yourself unable to gain perspective on life or if you feel overwhelmed and obsessing over whether the next pregnancy test will be positive or negative, then volunteer work is your remedy. Ask your intuitive guides to lead you to a place where your service is needed, and I promise you will be directed to the exact situation that you were meant to witness and participate in. Acts of kindness are free and do not depend on our economic, educational, or relationship status. Remembering that having a child is not a goal to be accomplished or a box to be checked off. A powerful act of love and service is important to facilitating the conception of your child as this practice will extend into motherhood. I like to refer to motherhood as my favorite volunteer work. It helps keep me honest and grounded in the essentials of what it is to be a human being.

Expectations, especially of motherhood and the idea of motherhood, are the most significant source of limiting beliefs. But it doesn't need to be that way. We do not need to look to events that have not occurred, and children we have not yet had, to begin to allow ourselves to live in the emotions and environment that our soul needs. The Law of Attraction suggests that you bring into your life what you are putting out. Practice being here and now, as the person you envision being once your child arrives. This will make the cosmic landing strip that much clearer for your child.

Once we get clear about what we want from parenthood, we can begin to analyze the thought patterns and beliefs that get in our way. Kate was a 37-year-old environmentalist and an advocate of sustainable living. She had a successful career as a writer and journalist and was an outspoken celebrity in her field. Her longtime partner was more than ready to have children; Kate had put it off for many years but wanted to do it before "it's too late."

As we began working together, I made it a point to start by asking the exact questions I asked you in this chapter. Kate was conscious of the fact that parenthood was hard, and she had some doubts about her ability to parent well. "It seems like even the best of parents still have problems with their kids. I'm afraid that I am just going to mess up my kids and pass on the trauma that I came from."

I see this pattern frequently, and while I understand it, the truth is that when we participate wholeheartedly in our own healing and model this behavior for our kids, it isn't necessary (or even possible) to be perfect. Our mere effort is enough to mitigate the biggest parenting issues. Kate had already done a lot of self-work. She had thought long and hard about the health of the Earth and human beings' role as its stewards and caretakers. As we continued to talk, I felt that Kate was avoiding voicing a more profound fear of pregnancy. And while all of her answers to my questions were relatively normal (in that she expected to find family and happiness from being a mom), her tone was flat and her expression of her excitement was unconvincing.

"Kate," I said, "remove your brain's interpretation of what I am asking you. Try and respond from the deepest, most internal space within, the space that you are afraid to put a voice to because it feels like if you voice it, it might become true."

She hesitated and sat for a few minutes. I could tell she was fighting her mind. Then she let out a huge, audible sigh and said, "I am afraid that the world is ending. I am afraid to bring a child to an Earth that is already overpopulated and running out of resources. I am afraid that I will not get pregnant because of this."

"Kate," I responded, "do you want to be a mother?"

"Yes," she said.

"Kate," I continued, "do you feel connected to a child out there who wants you to be his or her mother?"

"Yes!" she said, more emphatically.

"Good. I understand that your work must be so heart-wrenching, discouraging, and sad. I, too, see how the Earth has been underappreciated and cared for. I also see the problems that are facing us here, but what if, above your allegiance to help save the Earth, you had another, more significant, allegiance to your child?"

Her brain kicked in again. "But so many of my colleagues and scientists I know say the only way to save the Earth is to stop overpopulation. How can I go against what they say?"

I see this type of judgment far too often, and many limiting belief systems arise from the space in which we allow society's narrative to override our desire and knowing. So I asked Kate again to shift her allegiance to the spirit of her child. As she struggled with what that might mean for her work and belief system, many subsequent questions and insights arose. Many dealt with feeling overwhelmingly depressed and disheartened by the politics and state of fairness in the world.

I suggested that Kate take some time and write out what I call my Reasons Why exercise (see sidebar on page 102). This asks you to list on the left side of a page reasons you believe you are not able or should not have a child, such as the planet's overpopulation, difficulty in your relationship, or lack of financial stability. After that list is made, use the right side to list the reasons you should become a parent, including lots of love to give, a stable relationship, a loving family, etc. The only catch is that for every negative belief in the left column, you have to list two positive beliefs in the right column. So if you have ten reasons that you shouldn't, you must counter it with 20 reasons that you should. The reasons you should have a child then become part of a new belief pattern that is especially helpful to refer to when you are in a negative space.

Several weeks passed before Kate and I spoke again. I had thought about Kate often during that time. In so many ways, she represented the problematic conversation that many conscious and intelligent human beings are having at this moment in human history. We have access to so much data and knowledge, and we carry with us the capacity to feel empathy and compassion for other living beings, and yet so much suffering, despair, and inequality continue to thrive. Kate, having devoted her life to educating and bringing these issues to the forefront of people's awareness, occupied a challenging space—a space in which she was trying to positively impact the future, based on a dismal past. But in our follow-up conversation, I was surprised by the joy and lightness in her voice.

"I've switched my allegiance," she said proudly. "I'm ready to have my child."

"Amazing! What shifted for you over the last few weeks?" I asked.

"I remembered the happiest and most at peace that I ever felt was when I was an anthropology student studying tribes in South America. It's what inspired me to be an environmentalist. They had such joy and love in their community, and the children were so bright-eyed and happy. I think I have forgotten that I am a human being too, just like them—and that it's part of being human to want to have children and love them. And that is okay too, no matter what happens to the Earth."

Kate had eloquently stated something so beautiful and true. Her process to decide to have children was not at all haphazard. The limiting belief that she could not, and should not, have children because of the health of the planet had almost succeeded in blocking her pregnancy. She thought long and hard and finally chose allegiance with her son, who was born about a year later. From time to time, she drops me a line to tell me what a fantastic soul he is and how smart and compassionate he turned out to be. To which I always respond, "That is because he is here to help continue your work and save the Earth."

A little fact that I knew about him from the first conversation Kate and I shared.

## CULTIVATING AWARENESS OF THE NEGATIVE PEOPLE AND ENERGY IN OUR LIVES

As we work to identify where limiting beliefs are sourced, we often find the people and places that help prop up these views. No doubt you have experienced firsthand people who have extreme opinions about *your* fertility and reproductive health . . . and who often have no hesitation sharing their views with you.

Have you ever experienced being in a fabulous mood that quickly turned terrible after a conversation or interaction with someone else? Have you walked into a hotel room, restaurant, or friend's house, only to feel that something was off, so you turned around and left? Innate within all of us is a protective honing mechanism, a type of energetic security system that alerts us to people, places, and moments that can be dangerous and injurious to our being.

Your endocrine system is just one of the biological systems within your body that translates external threat into action. When you are experiencing hormonal shifts like those that occur around ovulation, PMS, or pregnancy, or as you are undergoing hormonal therapy in reproductive medicine, this energetic security system is on high alert. The human menstrual cycle is a dynamic process. The sex hormones—estrogen, testosterone, and progesterone— dramatically affect a woman's emotional state and her sexual desire. During ovulation, women's dreams often change, and their overall emotional state becomes more heightened.

From an evolutionary stance, your sensitivity with hormonal shifts can be seen as a physical response to identify and protect you from persons and environments that might endanger an implantation and pregnancy. My patients often describe experiences of heightened paranoia and sensitivity when it can be confusing and difficult to separate what is true from what is not. This is indeed something that many highly sensitive people have difficulty navigating once they begin to be more in touch with their intuition. Being tapped into your intuitive wisdom is freeing, but not always easy. Many people hide behind their rationalism, because living and expressing the world of feeling and sensing can be painful. A centuries-old legacy makes women innately understand the danger of being identified as intuitive. There remains an active force in the world working mainly through judgment, bullying, and ridicule to suppress that which it does not understand, or that which does not fit into popular opinion.

Most of the negative feedback I experience on social media is from people, unfortunately mostly women, who criticize the fact that I support my clients via unconventional and non–science-based methods. I had to move through my initial hurt, sadness, and defensiveness at these comments, and into a space where I no longer allowed myself to be impacted by their negativity. Ultimately, when I only allow in the energy and people who help my path to unfold in accord with universal law, I am unaffected by criticism. In many cases, I can be compassionate toward my critics and detractors, and understand that their judgments typically come from their trauma as human beings. Why else would someone be so adamant about what another human being does with his or her own body and reproduction?

Although there is a learning curve as you start to leave behind limiting beliefs and the fear that often caused them, doing so opens you up to a different and more honest way of life. In the long run, the more forthcoming we are with emotions and thoughts, the less likely we are to rely on gossip and judgmental rhetoric to protect our limited beliefs. When someone expresses a strong opinion that may or may not be at odds with your current psychological and emotional state, take a step back, bracket that opinion, and try to understand its context. Do not take it personally. Do not take it as law or fact, no matter how much social authority the person may have. Observe the reaction it elicits within you and bracket that too. Keep what resonates as applicable and perhaps "save the other for another day." Spiritual liberation often begins with liberation from language. This is a valuable skill to take into the terrain of spiritual fertility.

### Exercise: *Reasons Why*

I often recommend that this exercise be done with one's partner. It is a powerful tool for communication but requires the practice of compassionate listening. As your partner expresses his or her fears, remember that these are not directly about you; try not to take them personally.

Take out your journal or a piece of paper. On the left side of a page, list the reasons you believe you are not able or should not have a child (the planet's overpopulation, difficulty in your relationship, lack of financial stability, and so on). Then, on the right side of the page, detail the reasons you should become a parent (lots of love to give, a stable relationship, a loving family, etc.). The only catch is that for every negative belief in the left column, you have to list *two* positive beliefs in the right column. So if you have 10 reasons that you shouldn't have a child, you must counter it with 20 reasons that you should. The reasons you should have a child then become part of a new belief pattern that is especially helpful to refer to when you are feeling negative. Place your list around your home in a prominent place, so you can be reminded of it throughout the day.

## CHOOSING WORDS AND BELIEF SYSTEMS

For many, it is difficult to speak about something we want but haven't yet experienced, such as pregnancy, that can only be conceptualized through what we have learned socially and culturally. The narrative that circulates in society influences the experiences that people have within it. The words and belief systems of those around us tend to affect us, especially when those words resonate with our deepest fears.

Through mindfulness, we can cultivate an awareness of the people and energy in our lives that feel negative and make us doubt the intuitive knowledge of our body. I stress that even the freedom to enter into conversation with your reproductive choice to have a baby is in and of itself revolutionary. For many, this revolution has not yet occurred. If you have been fortunate to be born now in the right place with the freedom to choose if and when you would like to have a child, then remember to hold this as a sacred privilege. You are a frontier person, and frontier people are always the bravest. Act with courage. Avoid fear. Construct new paradigms for the planet and examine the limiting beliefs that keep you from growing. Show our repressive history and the oppressive holdouts on the Earth what free sexuality and a free uterus look like. Help us to evolve out of—not devolve into—replacing fallen structures with new masters like modern medicine and cultural materialism.

Stories of early-onset infertility, recurrent miscarriage, and traumatic births might seem like full disclosure by doctors and medical systems that feel obliged to present all possible outcomes. However, even hypothesizing about an individual's potential fertility or infertility can have a hypnotizing impact. It can be a destabilizing force, and at times, can even manifest infertility. The stories we hear from childhood into adulthood influence what we understand and how we connect to our sexuality and our reproductive capacity. The subtle energetics that influence the endocrine system respond to negative, stress-induced emotional beliefs.

Look more deeply into the unconscious ways in which your connection to reproduction is influenced by the social, medical, and familial narratives that we sometimes blindly share and perpetuate. There is no one individual cause of infertility, and no individual is the cause of the infertility she might experience. The way each of us represents and extends our unique freedom, alongside the beliefs that we choose to hold, helps support all people on the planet. It helps liberate us and creates a better future for all children, not just the ones we choose to create.

## Spiritual Fertility Essentials

Our beliefs, whether we are conscious of them or not, greatly influence our actions. Deep beliefs that might be hidden under layers of shame and guilt are often difficult to unearth and express, and those held by society can also impact an individual's growth. In this chapter, we explored how, by developing intuition, you become better equipped to question the convictions from which you and society are operating. Just as positive beliefs can balance and calm the nervous system, limiting ones can engage and disturb the balance of your system. These limiting beliefs sabotage all other work you might be doing, even practices that are rooted in psychology and spirituality.

You can unearth your own doubts about becoming a parent and apply the tools offered here for alchemizing these beliefs into insight and clarity. By posing difficult questions—especially about possible regrets and changes in your relationship—instead of granting those fears power, you instead gain the ability to transform them. When you examine what it is that you are looking to feel when you become a parent and start to practice embodying these energetics, you change your frequency and your reality.

# Chapter 6

# The Unconscious as Healer

I believe the ultimate goal of self-care is creating the space to hear the whispers of your higher self; often, these whispers can be heard in your dreams.

We all dream. In our dreams, we have access to the deep well of collective thought and memory. Some dreams, remembered or not, take place in the dark stillness of nighttime. Just as it can be difficult to capture in words the language and messages delivered in the unconscious space of the dream, it can prove challenging to find appropriately descriptive language for working with the unconscious. Complex and hard-to-explain theories about the nature of the universe, intuition, and how to trust in the flow of cosmic timing can begin in simple, easy-to-integrate practices. Most of these practices start with opening a space for listening to the quiet voice within.

The moments between the unconscious dream world and the conscious waking world hold great value for accessing thoughts, emotions, and messages from our higher self. Creating a practice to listen to these messages can be simple but sets the foundation for a life led by intuition. The dream world itself can be rich in imagery, so rich that an entire study has been formulated to help translate these symbolic themes. Dream interpretation seeks to draw out deeper desires, fears, longings, and blockages that might be keeping you from connecting to your mind and spirit, and from hearing the universal messages intended just for you.

There is a rich lineage throughout history of messages delivered through dreams regarding events that will occur, people the dreamer will meet, and children the dreamer will have. On my intake form I ask my clients about birth- and pregnancy-related dreams right alongside questions about their menstrual cycle. I know that dreams are just as important as vital medical information when it comes to understanding the whole picture of a person's fertility health.

The Bible contains more than 20 stories of heavenly messages delivered through dreams. In Hindu sacred texts, multiple stories share prophecies that appeared in the unconscious space of the dream. Many ancient traditions viewed messages sent in dreams as significant information from the universe worthy of interpretation. Indeed, the richness and depth that a dream can hold, especially to those with vivid intuitive gifts, can sometimes feel indistinguishable from reality. Setting an intention with your unconscious creates a path for information to be delivered through the highway of your dreamscape. This can be beneficial when trying to relinquish strong attachments to an outcome, such as achieving pregnancy. Receiving and listening to the messages of the unconscious can provide an infrastructure of trust, allowing you to relax and be less vigilant.

Sometimes it can feel isolating and lonely when you don't have a clear vision or connection to the spirit of your child. And while it is not necessary to have this connection to become pregnant, I believe it is possible when you are given the right tools, and space to listen. Just like the characters and personalities in our own lives, some voices are louder than others. This applies to the spirits of our children, as well.

Some spirits are quite gregarious and present, while others are more introverted and reverent. I encourage my clients not to be discouraged if they cannot connect, but to instead allow this "blockage" to set up a line of inquiry and investigation. It is not uncommon to unearth strong and clear relationships to future children once you begin to listen to the language of the unconscious. The unconscious speaks through the universal imagery of dreams, synchronicity, and symbols.

By the end of the next few chapters, you will know how to speak the basic language of the unconscious. As a reminder, the most powerful tool that transcends all languages and connects directly to your child's spirit is that of unconditional love. Allow yourself to move without critical judgment of how good you are at dreaming, catching the magic of everyday synchronicity, or summoning up lullabies. Loving our future children without the conditions that we impose on ourselves is the most powerful of all energetic tools.

## LISTENING TO THE UNCONSCIOUS

As children, we learn the great myths of our world. Fairy tales, myths, and fables all share the common journey of a single character, or hero, through adverse environments that threaten the hero's core beliefs in self and other.

These themes are related through larger-than-life monsters and symbolic creatures or whimsical landscapes. The Hero's Journey is a common motif in cross-cultural narratives; this is a framework in which individuals embark on a quest, through which they learn a profound life lesson about their own nature and the nature of humankind.

Think of your dreams as your own mythic journey that uses the exact type of rich imagery as the stories of old. But just as you had to pay attention to story time as a child, you must also pay attention to the dream to fully grasp its ultimate message.

Several tools can help with this. I have found that sometimes the more difficult part of listening to the messages my clients receive is believing in them. Again, the power of the conscious mind to override the rich landscape of all other perceptions is a hallmark of modern life. It can be scary to listen to feelings and thoughts that don't fit into the reality in which you are living. And painfully, many people, even those who love you the dearest, will question the validity of what you "know" from a developed conversation with the unconscious.

However, if there were ever a language through which you could communicate with the spirit of your unborn child, it exists in the tender, vulnerable space of the unconscious. Ultimately, it is your duty to yourself to stand by your individual wisdom. There is never a need to defend, rationalize, or explain your understanding to anyone who questions it, unless you choose to do so. For many, the defense of the intuitive and unconscious world becomes a call to arms and life path in and of itself. For others, some of whom you would never suspect of living by intuitive wisdom, nothing ever need be said or done to declare their findings.

## Exercise: *Dream Journal*

Many people have spoken of the power of writing first thing in the morning in the liminal space when you are closest to sleep, halfway between the conscious and unconscious world. A dream journal is a powerful tool for connecting and communicating with the spirit of your child and your ancestors. Dreams present us with a set of symbols that we are able to decode. The dream world has direct access to the collective unconscious; therefore, you can ask a question in a dream and receive guidance from universal intelligence.

I structure my dream journal exercise a little differently from most people. I ask that you write a specific question in your dream journal before you go to sleep and meditate on this question as you drift into the night. First thing in the morning, whether you remember your dreams or not, answer the question as quickly as possible. Write it down, regardless of whether or not it makes sense. After you answer the question, you can draw, describe, or record your memories from your dreams. Look for imagery that stands out, such as ancestors, animals, buildings, or oceans and rivers. Interpret your own dream in your journal before asking others what they think. And if you do have a visitation from the spirit of your child in a dream, keep it safe and protected until your child is conceived and you are in your second trimester. A dream is a space where spirit is incubated to be born into reality, so too much attention too soon can be disrespectful to the artistic process and threaten the masterpiece.

I learned from a powerful shaman with whom I studied in my early years that the ultimate power in healing others comes down to a simple statement: "Do I act, or do I not act?" I have come to understand that in personal healing, this translates to: "Do I ask and listen, or do I not?"

One choice impacts the energies that are at work with a declarative force and vision, while the other recedes into the calm nonparticipant, who allows the situation to play out in accord with the universe. Both statements acknowledge that each of us is connected to a larger self, and when we are in need of cosmic support, we can ask for it through the landscape of our dreams. I asked for such support in my own path to motherhood.

## THE MESSAGES FROM THE DREAM

I was ready, or at least I thought I was ready, to have a child at age 26. Having known about my daughter's presence for over a decade, I wanted to meet her in real life. I had found a loving relationship with my husband, set up a successful private practice, and healed many injuries from my past. But the timing was not right, and the next years brought into my life a doctorate, a residency in China, relocation of home, and further deepening of my practice in healing infertility for others.

*You can't rush a masterpiece,* I said to myself again and again.

By age 32, the longing to become a mother turned into anxiety and fear that it would not happen. Looking back now, 32 seems so young, but the combination of being strongly connected to my daughter's spirit, while helping person after person to have their own healthy and happy babies, raised doubt for me in the universe, my partner, and my path. My desire and my impatience were becoming an issue in my relationship and put me into a state of fear that something was amiss with my fertility and health. I began to convince myself that it would take forever to get pregnant once I began to try. Something had to shift.

One February morning, thick in the winter blues and my sadness, I was standing on the subway platform when a whisper from my highest self directed me to a popular yoga studio in Manhattan for a 10  meditation class. As many of you know, one of the hardest things to do when you are down is drag yourself to the very activities that will help you. I hadn't been to yoga in months, and I had never been to this particular studio. The teacher was a sage who had been a practitioner of yoga his entire 60-plus years on the planet. I sat in deep meditation as he directed us to imagine calling back into our bodies all the various energies and selves that we projected into the world. He asked us to consolidate all the energy that we expended on anxiety and worry and to seal it back inside our hearts. It was a beautiful meditation that made me capable of listening to my higher self in a clearer and more profound way.

That night, before I closed my eyes, I asked my guides and the Divine itself to offer me some clarity about my fertility through a dream. I prayed that I would listen to and receive the message, no matter the outcome. The symbols and messages I received in the following dream were so powerful that my anxiety was obliterated and my trust in cosmic timing was reinforced.

In this dream, my husband and I were swimming off the southern coast of South Africa, illuminated by a full moon. We were united and close as we noticed a small airplane with an open door circling in the sky above. Someone was trying to parachute out of the plane into the ocean below. They could not jump because there was something blocking their landing spot in the water. In the dream, we spotted two huge humpback whales circling below the plane and sky jumper, and we realized that we had to do something to help. We swam out and each wrestled a whale to the side of a huge rock that jetted up from the waves. Just as we did this, the parachuter floated to Earth, landing gently in the water, safe and sound despite the delay.

In many systems of dream interpretation, the whale is related to ancestors. This dream showed me that my partner and I were not only capable of setting aside the influences of our family origins but that, as we did so, we were creating the pathway for our daughter to be born. The literal metaphor of someone parachuting to Earth describes someone being incarnated and born. The dream healed me; the next morning, I awoke without any anxiety or worry as to when I would meet my daughter. I simply knew that as long as I was next to my husband and we were swimming together, it was going to happen.

I became pregnant four months later, and by using the tools of unconscious and conscious conception, it happened quickly. Our beautiful daughter was born under a triple water astrological sign of the fish (whale reference) in an unbroken amniotic sack, the caul, just as the dream had predicted: under the moonlight and ruled by water.

Even though this was a powerfully healing dream, I still had to make a choice to believe in it. Such is true of all our encounters in life, both positive and negative. We have to practice emotional maturity, especially when we are most triggered and challenged by our emotions. We also have to practice trusting in the infrastructure of the universe and take steps to expose our innermost hurt and shadow to something that is beyond our control. Vulnerability and softening can create the space needed for healing to occur. When we do this, when we finally allow our spiritual guides in, our higher selves and the part of our being that is infinite, we are often given a suitcase that contains the maps by which to walk through our despair and disbelief. You can find your way through without this help, but receiving help is essential to being a modern-day parent, and often one of the earliest lessons of motherhood.

## DREAMS AS PROPHECY

Dreams link the conscious to the unconscious. Dreams have access to the well of universal wisdom that we all participate within but cannot see clearly in our day-to-day lives. There is so much wisdom and guidance in a dream. All you need do is ask and listen.

My intake form asks people if they have ever dreamed of their future child. Some people laugh, some people just skip it altogether, and some list detailed dreams stretching back for years. Kim was about 32 weeks pregnant when I asked her, "Do you have an instinct about when your baby will be born?"

"Not exactly an instinct," she said, "but I had a dream that he would be born on January 10th."

I was not at all surprised when, on January 9th, I received a text message that said that Kim was on the way to the hospital.

I started to study the prophetic nature of dreams years ago. I had been sitting in an integrative gynecology class that weekend, next to a brilliant woman named Uma. Uma spoke five languages, practiced Chinese medicine, was a Taoist scholar, wrote operas, and had two beautiful children, among many other accomplishments. During a break, I leaned over and said, "Uma, I had the strangest dream last night that I had a huge tattoo of a dragon on my lower abdomen. It was so beautiful."

"Ahhhh," she responded matter-of-factly, "well, that just means you are going to have a baby in the year of the dragon."

And as simply as that, she helped me divine the message of the dream. My daughter was born in the year of the dragon, a sign that indicates longevity and good health.

## THE LINK BETWEEN YOUR
## UNCONSCIOUS AND YOUR WOMB

The very first traditional Chinese medicine class that I sat in many years ago began by describing the two major forces that are at work on the planet and in our bodies. Dr. Shen described yang as active, masculine, functional, bright, warm, dominating daytime and the sun. Yin, he said, was receptive, feminine, dark, cooling, and at its strongest during the night and the light of the moon. These two principles are forever seeking balance with each other and are a part of the continued creative and destructive process of the human reproductive cycle. The uterus is classified as a yin organ, but it contains the principles of creation and destruction, yin and yang, and both masculine and feminine qualities. In a nutshell, the uterus is a universe. Its sacred and receptive space holds a space very similar to the landscape of the dream.

Each of our gestations takes place within a uterus. The time it takes to incubate is marked by developmental stages of growth that we often count through weeks and trimesters. But spiritually, many other important seeds are also taking root during this time. Within the womb, we connect to the countless ancestors who came before us. We are also able to connect to the dimensions of consciousness that we lose access to once we are born. It takes some time for this loss of access to occur. Young infants still live very much between the two worlds of the conscious and unconscious, continuing to sleep most of the day and staying disengaged from the waking world. With time and the intake of the food, air, and beauty of Earth, each of our unique spirits incarnates deeper and deeper into the flesh. Our rational minds are at the helm of what we categorize as real, while the memory of the numinous recedes into the space of the dream and the unconscious. Some children can still recount incredible details of the past lives that they lived. Others can recall in words the specifics of the nature of the universe, God, and the meaning of life.

The experiences that we have with wombs in our lifetimes—including being birthed from them and containing our children in the uterus during pregnancy—are clear examples of the womb's capacity to merge with the other. The term *other* is used to describe the energies of the people, places, and phenomena that we categorize as different from us and existing outside of us. We often place people into this category when we are unsure, threatened, or afraid. This defensive and protective instinct can happen when there is trauma, or unwelcomed and insulting energy, but more fundamentally, we often seek to define the other when we are afraid. Fear creates many types of walls energetically, and sometimes those invisible walls turn into real ones.

The space of the uterus is meant to reflect the space of the unconscious. It is meant to be open and to communicate and translate the deep mirroring that it shares with the universe. The womb models the cycles of death and regeneration that we all face. Unfortunately, we often lose the wisdom of the unconscious with the development of ego and with the passing of time.

Just before I sat down to write this, I fell very hard onto a strip of ice that I did not see. I was afraid that I had hurt myself badly. The trauma of a past fall I experienced many years ago came rushing back. I cried, but because I was with my daughter, I tried to pull myself together as quickly as possible. The first fall I experienced two decades prior had been at the beginning of my sexual exploration with the world. It very literally occurred as I followed my boyfriend down a hiking path that I knew to be deteriorated from heavy rains. I fell a good 10 feet, hurting my back because I listened to him instead of to my instinct. But I was trying so hard to win his love through sexuality and physicality, and because I was so new at the game of love, I had very little knowledge of how to play. He was cruel and careless with my feelings, and that fall, away from him, was my unconscious loudly telling me to listen to the signs and take a different path.

The fear I felt while slipping on the ice reminded me of the deep lack of control that so many people experience when trying to conceive. I felt mad and angry that when I allowed my consciousness to slip for a single minute, I hurt myself. I ended up being just fine, but the real message of the ice slip was the reminder that even as I write and describe what it means to connect to the unconscious, its real power (and indeed, the reason we should respect it) comes through the symbolic events and actions of our lives. We too easily forget that—just as the uterus can open and contract to contain life—reality itself is on far more of a continuum than we acknowledge.

So much of the hypervigilance we give to the details of charting, ovulation kits, lab results, and perfectly timed sex is rooted in fear. None of us likes to slip on the ice, and none of us likes to feel vulnerable. When we see trauma approaching us, we defend against it. We make split-second decisions to protect ourselves from what we see coming.

My friend, who comes from a lineage of great explorers, once told me of a paragliding accident she had in the mountains of New Mexico. After jumping and hitting a boulder, her helmet came off, which in paragliding can mean certain death; however, in the moments before she barreled into a second rock, she threw her arm out to defend her more vulnerable organs and screamed at the top of her lungs as she impacted. She shattered her arm but survived.

"Why did this accident occur? What was its importance in the way your life unfolded?" I asked her. This wise, brave explorer of the Amazon jungle responded, "At that moment, I trusted authority more than I trusted my own instinct and knowledge. I knew it was a sketchy situation, but I listened to the authority of the instructor instead of myself. That was the ultimate lesson of that accident."

If we respect our slips, falls, illnesses, and losses, and take into account the deeper message from our unconscious that these moments in our life present, we will learn how to lower our defensive walls and live a less guarded and less fearful life.

## TRUSTING YOUR UNCONSCIOUS

Trusting your unconscious can sometimes feel like trusting in God. The more disillusion, suffering, and trauma that you live through, the harder it is to feel there is anything out there paying attention to your well-being. I often hear from people that they were once optimistic, positive, and trusting, but the loss of a baby and denied motherhood had worn them down into harder, and more clinical, disbelievers.

One of my first duties to this type of broken person is to remind my patient of her primary and essential relationship to the Divine and the mystical, and to help her reengage with a trust in the universe. Once you have lost your faith in the infrastructure of the universe, you cannot rebuild that trust overnight. And the common tools that are available to those who have not walked through the shadowlands of grief just do not work.

Many people are critical and cynical of spiritual work because spiritual work has failed to provide them with the correct language and tools to excavate their souls. Most gurus thrive on light and feel-good endorphins, and easily dismiss the person in the crowd who questions their authority as an unenlightened and immature soul. In contrast, I love working with the spiritually cynical. The success I have experienced leading them through baby steps back to trusting in the universe is instrumental for many of their successful pathways to a healthy pregnancy and birth. The best way to help individuals build their trust in the Divine is by assisting them in developing their awareness of the unconscious.

Lauren had been trying to conceive for many years. She was still young at 31, and therefore had decided to give it time before using IVF and reproductive medicine. She lived in a community of New Age spiritual people to which she'd first been drawn a decade earlier. Although incredibly supportive of women's health and empowerment, they were also, as she described, extremely judgmental in their practice of "woo-woo." She had been through several different types of healers, psychics, and therapists, all of whom suggested they knew why she was not conceiving. But as the years passed, her original faith was degraded by her observations of the community that she lived within. She saw hypocrisy within their ethics and morals, and she began to withdraw from her friends. I sensed in Lauren a broken relationship to the universe, and via e-mail she warned me that she didn't respond well to spiritual and energetic work. She had built a wall.

When people wish to work with me and make the claim that they don't believe in the "spiritual stuff," this is always a good sign to me that they actually *do*—and that somehow, along the way, they lost their faith. The powerful tool of disengaging and falling back into trust and receptivity cannot occur when we are defensive and critical of our potential to experience the phenomenon of spirit.

In American law, we put the burden of proof on the court, allowing the accused to defend their case until proven guilty. Once an injury to faith has occurred, as it did for Lauren, a person begins to live like everyone is guilty until proven innocent. This amount of prosecution is exhausting, and more than that, it requires a person to live in an actively vigilant fashion. When we cannot trust the universe around us, we cannot rest in the receptive and relaxed body necessary for conception. Lauren needed tools to remember not what she had once believed, but something that dwelled even deeper, beyond her lost practice. She needed a new relationship with God.

I asked Lauren to begin a synchronicity journal (see sidebar on page 123): a running list of details that I compared to Nancy Drew's detective notebook. I asked her to write down connections that she saw in her environment, such as catching a glimpse of a cardinal sitting on her doorstep, and later that day sitting at a restaurant that had cardinals on the wallpaper. Another example could be hearing an old favorite song just before getting a call from the friend who had introduced her to it, or taking a different route to work and bumping into a loved one. When rebuilding faith, baby steps are essential. Lauren didn't need anyone to tell her to believe in the universe; she needed the universe to show her that it was, in fact, all around her—and that it believed in her.

Small steps and practices can grow into significant pathways to wisdom. Had I not listened to the small voice that suggested I head to meditation, I probably would not have had the dream that cured me of anxiety about my daughter's birth. Offerings that we make when we are at our most vulnerable can be the scariest ones. But even if you fall, you will be okay. Quite possibly, the slip will lead you to a crucial soul lesson.

## Exercise: *Synchronicity Journal*

When rebuilding faith, baby steps are essential. A synchronicity journal allows the universe to show you that it is all around you and that it believes in you.

Create a running list of details you observe in your environment. Envision a detective as she pulls a notebook out of her pocket to record important facts. Write down connections that you see in your environment, such as catching a glimpse of a cardinal sitting on your doorstep, and later that day sitting at a restaurant with cardinals on the wallpaper. Other examples could be hearing an old favorite song just before getting a call from the friend who introduced you to it, or taking a different route to work and bumping into a loved one. Choose any journal to record these messages. I often text myself the synchronicities I observe, or I record them in my calendar.

A synchronicity journal is powerful magic that is grounded in observational science. I have seen this exercise make even the staunchest rationalist smile with curiosity and joy. It is also a wonderful exercise for deepening your connection to your guides.

## Spiritual Fertility Essentials

The moments between the unconscious dream world and the conscious waking world hold great value for accessing thoughts, emotions, and messages from our higher self. Creating a practice to listen to these messages can be simple but sets the foundation for a life led by intuition.

Determining the messages from your unconscious can be like decoding a mysterious map full of symbols and strange imagery that is still somehow very familiar. Your intuitive guidance knows how to navigate your unconscious far better than your analytical mind.

In this chapter, we discovered the rich history and tradition of messages about pregnancy and future children being delivered through dreams. You learned how the womb is symbolic of the unconscious and how dream interpretation theories were modeled after theories of how consciousness develops during gestation. While many experts might suggest they know what your dream's message means, your own intuitive wisdom is ultimately the best translator of the symbols that show up for you. It is easy to lose the wisdom of the unconscious to the ego. We often miss the messages we were intended to receive because we are busy protecting ourselves from vulnerability. But the message continues to find a way to show up in our lives. When you practice observing the symbolic events and actions in your life, you gain insight into the powerful tool of trusting yourself.

# Chapter 7

# Symbols, Synchronicity, and Cosmic Timing

There is a science to observing intuition, and it can be a methodical undertaking with a purpose, procedure, operation, and conclusion. Learning to listen to the unconscious allows us a window into the magic that is all around us. The unconscious can link each of our unique beings with the grand collective that governs us all. Faith may well be the evidence of things unseen, as the New Testament suggests, but I don't think that it has to be. The rich symbols that surround us in daily life, and that capture our attention through synchronicity, are a different kind of proof in the unseen cosmic infrastructure. Pausing to acknowledge these proofs can map a path forward for each of us. If and when we need encouragement—especially when we are in the essential moments of our lives, be it choosing new directions, closing past chapters, or listening to the call of our spirits for radical change—symbols, synchronicity, and cosmic timing can provide us with confirmation that we are, indeed, on the correct trajectory.

All of us are connected to symbols, even when we are not aware of them. Symbolism around names conveys a lot of information before we even meet. Just think of the times when you are introduced to someone and think that they don't *seem* like their given name, or that they should be called something different. Names are intimately tied to our identity, and we are extremely tied to identity in Western culture. We have access to a collective and unified consciousness on Earth, but we continue to cling to dualism and individuality as the truth. In traditional Asian cultures of old, people introduced themselves by leading with their family name before their first name, a nod to the idea of being stronger as a group than as an individual. In the West, our individuality is very much an indicator of our success and we are often only known by our first names.

However, there are limits to identifying with your sense of individual self. What is known in psychology and philosophy as *the transpersonal* is the important study of examining states of consciousness beyond personal identity. Exploring the transpersonal allows each of us to study the ways in which our individual psychology and consciousness are a reflection of the whole, and vice versa. Carl Jung, one of the founders of transpersonal psychology, developed numerous techniques of incorporating mystical spiritual traditions into the clinical setting. He developed the concepts of symbols, synchronicity, and cosmic timing as the language of the unconscious. All three of these are important to take into account when understanding the complete picture of each individual patient and their symptoms. As we have discussed, the multiple pathways that set the foundation for incarnation and birth are inclusive of the whole of a family's history, the energetic state of the world, and the secrets of the unconscious.

The magic and messages of the universe are meant to be comforting and validating when you feel isolated and alone. They reveal the ways that you as an individual are still connected to phenomena beyond a singular and isolated life. When you are experiencing major life transitions, it is not uncommon to see the messages all around you . . . if you take the time to notice. For instance, more than a year before I sat down to write this very chapter, I was standing on a street corner in Los Angeles. I looked over and noticed that I was standing right next to fashion designer and women's advocate Diane von Furstenberg. What was strange is that I felt like I knew her; she was intimately familiar to me. It was a highly creative and magical time in my own life, as I made new soul agreements about expanding my work of spiritual fertility into the world. A year later, almost to the day, as I began this chapter on synchronicity, I received a call from Diane von Furstenberg's office inviting me to work with her. The sense of familiarity I had on that street corner was a premonition of a future path. Moments like these are designed to support your faith. They are exhilarating and uplifting, and enhance a certain feeling of connectivity and purpose.

Outside of the comfort that unconscious signals can provide, they have an even more powerful and transformative impact. When you begin to live your life listening to and trusting the messages from your most interior self, you begin to dismantle the power that you have given to other people, especially those in authority. Each step you take to shift the power dynamic away from the exterior world, and everything you do to stop looking outside of yourself for the answers, empowers your own realization that you already have access to all that you are seeking.

When we break away from tribalism and monotheistic cultures, we transfer the power once attributed to God to those who claim they have the power of God. Kings, presidents, and doctors are the new placeholders to comfort our fear and anxiety. We miss out on a huge opportunity when we look to others to fix our sadness, illness, infertility, and confusion. If we continue to refabricate the broken systems of old, we will never return to the harmony and equality that once ruled this planet. Simply connecting to intuitive wisdom might not provide enough of a catalyst to change the politics and disagreements of Earth, but it can remind and reassure each of us, individually, of our collectivity and ultimate connection.

Here are some examples of meaningful symbols, synchronicity, and cosmic timing:

- Experiencing déjà vu, or the feeling of having seen or heard something before

- Receiving a call from a friend shortly after thinking of the person

- Sensing precognition about falling in love or marrying someone in your first meeting

- Picking up on messages from animals

- Observing astrological occurrences such as full moons, new moons, and equinoxes

- Being asked the same question by several different people, such as, "What is your astrological sign?"

- Overhearing conversations that are about exactly what you are thinking of in the moment

The individual path of spiritual connection and actualization is revolutionary. Its power to comfort you in sadness and grief can be exponentially grown into an alchemical classroom, where questions about your deep issues of this lifetime are answered. A dream can show you your child's face or a map of how to heal your greatest fear. A moment of synchronistic connection with a stranger can deliver a catalyzing moment when you give yourself permission to follow a different path, love, or career. A lunar eclipse can summon a deep memory of lust and desire that reminds you of your life purpose.

Many people argue that we are ultimately alone as individuals on the Earth, especially as we have moved farther and farther away from community. We are unique and highly spiritual creatures, tied to a global collective that has existed for a very long time. Your children's children will see proof of this interconnectedness, which all began with a simple message delivered to you at present, most likely through your unconscious.

## STEPPING INTO SYNCHRONICITY

Choosing to have a child is *big*. The more aware and present you have been in your own life, the more intense of a decision it can be, even when you have a socially accepted support system of spouse, family, and career. Fear can grow when you remove just one of these factors. I've worked with many people over the years who struggled with making this choice, not because of a lack of desire or a lack of trust in the call to be a parent, but because they were missing something they felt society told them they needed to have—such as a partner, financial stability, or extended family.

The latter was true of Tatiana, who had immigrated away from her one surviving relative decades ago. Tatiana's partner was also an only child from a broken and dismantled family. Together they both had the desire to start a family but hesitated; they knew that if anything happened to them, there would be no one left to care for their child and little money to help. As we were exploring her fear and preparing the way for pregnancy during one of our sessions, Tatiana said, "I dreamt of my grandmother last night. She was so close that I could smell her perfume and feel her warm breath on my cheek. I was so sad when I woke up. She's not here."

"But she is," I responded. "That was her telling you that she is here for not only you but for your future child too."

"I want to believe that," she replied. "I mean, I *do* believe that, but I've been fighting and struggling on my own for so long." For many people, the desire to live a more spiritual life is very much present, but often, the armor that they have had to put on to survive reflects faith away instead of allowing it in.

"How did you meet John?" I asked.

Her energy shifted and lightened. "We met at our friend's dinner party. I knew I loved him the first time we spoke. We were both running late and met in the elevator on the way up. It was meant to be." As she said the last sentence, she figured out why I had asked her this question.

"Is choosing to have a child just like that, something you know in your heart?"

"Yes, it often is." I smiled back.

After a pause, Tatiana said, "I don't know if I'm right or if I'm just saying this because it makes me feel better, but I think I was meant to have a child the moment I stepped into that elevator with John. I'm going to trust in that power over my fear, and I'm going to trust that he and I are not really alone."

Tatiana overcame the lineage of her isolated, fractured, and displaced history; instead of focusing on the ways she'd survived without anyone's help, she chose to recognize the unseen support of the universe, which had been with her all along.

So often, the signs and timing are already present in a person's life, but what is lacking is the permission to give these events credit and acknowledge their power. Many people in our lives will be supportive and encouraging when we share the stories about magical moments, while others will quickly turn their own cynicism toward us with a vengeance. I've learned the hard way that the more triggered and defensive a person is when you share information about alternative practices (such as holistic medicine, astrology, intuition, and synchronicity), the more this is a result of that person's own trauma. I tell my clients it's best not to try and change these staunch opinions, but to instead send those individuals as much unconditional love as you can. Maintain allegiance to your observations of such phenomena as a way of communicating with the spirit of your unborn child, and save the energy you would expend on arguing for something else, like growing a baby!

## Exercise: *Fertility Altar*

Creating a fertility altar is one of my favorite tools of spiritual fertility. This simple exercise is rooted in feng shui, an ancient system of interior design that describes the way that our home reflects the energetics of our life.

Can you make space in your life and your home, and by extension, for a child? Select an area of your home that feels peaceful and that you can easily see. Many people use the top of a dresser or a small side table as a base, although some make mobiles or bulletin boards the focus of their altar. I suggest adding the fertility symbols that you observe in your life, such as a picture of a family tree that you played on as a child, or images of your ancestors to whom you feel a positive attachment. In feng shui, fire is contraindicated in the space that reflects fertility, as fire is a great cleansing force that is powerful for clearing energy out but not necessarily for inviting energy to settle in. I suggest flowers, incense (which connects the earth to heaven through smoke), and music. Most importantly, spend time with your altar daily as a space to connect to your child's spirit.

### MESSAGES FROM YOUR CHILD'S SPIRIT

My client Ann had a different kind of faith in the universe to test, especially because the choice she would make to become a mother using IVF and donor sperm has been the path of so few women throughout history. Increasingly, I have been honored to work with this new type of mother whom I call the frontier woman because she is on the forefront of redefining the pathway to motherhood.

For centuries, the establishment of marriage was required to have children, but as women have gained footing in the economy and finally have the chance to be truly financially sovereign, we are discovering new ways to become mothers. Ann was a successful New York City executive. She had been a lifelong athlete and was highly educated about her own body and the spiritual connection between mind and body. She had made the decision in her late 30s to freeze her eggs, wanting to take the pressure off of getting pregnant not only for herself but potential partners.

The irony of developing your career in Western culture as a woman is that the thousands of hours you have to work to succeed almost always consumes the height of your reproductive years. It's not the same for men. By the time most women are in a place where they will not be passed over for a promotion because they took off a year to have a child or needed leave because of pregnancy-related complications, they are usually in their 40s.

I have said time and time again that older mothers make the best mothers, and I stand by that sentiment. A woman who has experienced both the good and bad of the world, and who has had the time to develop her own interests, passions, and desires before motherhood, brings to her child a wealth of wisdom—and often, a level of financial security to help foster her child's creativity and education.

I also want to make it extremely clear that I do not believe in the strict age categories that Western reproductive medicine places on women's fertility. While I ultimately support each individual's choice to freeze eggs earlier in their reproductive years, I have seen many cases where having frozen eggs was either completely unnecessary or too heavily relied on, especially when those eggs were not fertilized upon retrieval. It is important to take the time to listen to your instincts. I have developed an entire ritual process for egg freezing that I call Always Connected. It can provide comfort and spiritual support for not only you but also your eggs and embryos as you go through the fertility process. At the center of the ritual is holding a space for unconditional love, both for yourself and your future children.

I have seen unconditional love make all the difference. It certainly made a difference in Ann's fertility process. Several years after her decision to freeze her eggs, she found herself being loudly called by her child's spirit. She knew it was time and had confidence in her ability to be an excellent mother. However, she still had to grapple with some difficult decisions as a "single mother by choice." The women I have personally worked with in this category are in their 30s and 40s and extremely clear that they are prepared for motherhood, with or without a partner. For many, the allure of using a donor for sperm allows them to remove the variable of having to first find a life partner. In today's world, where so many potential partners already have children from previous relationships, the notion of being a single mother is no longer stigmatized. Ann felt the pull of her child's spirit so strongly that she seamlessly moved beyond the fear that often comes from being at the forefront of a movement.

There were some comforting signs and signals from the universe that showed its support along the way. I often describe this feeling to my clients by saying, "Imagine that your life is a marathon; as you run, there will be people along the way shouting their support and there will be banners held high, encouraging you. Look for them, especially if you need support or have lost your route."

One such banner of universal support came as Ann and I were taking a walk after her session. We had been speaking about her awareness of her baby's spirit and about how she felt she was almost ready to start trying to become pregnant when we turned a corner in New York's SoHo district to find a very special message intended for her.

Art can play a major role in delivering universal messages. Just as Ann said the words "I think I'm ready," she spotted a small ziplock bag taped to a building's wall. It was a gift from a New York City graffiti artist who places "free art" around the city. When she picked it up, we discovered that it was a breathtakingly beautiful drawing of a baby's face. I had chills as I said to her, "That's for you, Ann, take it."

"You're right, it is for me," she responded as she slipped the bag into her purse. Ann conceived on the first round of IVF a few months later and had a fantastically healthy pregnancy and birth. Her little girl is beautiful and strong, and experiences nothing but love from her mother and her mother's community. I never doubted Ann's capacity to healthily conceive and carry, but for much of the world, one additional fact about Ann would elicit fear and unnecessary judgment: Ann was 47 when her daughter was born.

## Exercise: *Always Connected*

Several years ago, when women began to freeze their eggs years before they were ready to begin conceiving, I was asked to develop a ritual to help make the process more sacred.

At first, I recommended the lullaby ritual (see page 65); this was helpful but didn't feel celebratory or joyful enough. Around that time, my wedding anniversary occurred and we, like many others, had saved some of our wedding cake in the freezer to eat later. I started recommending to my clients that they buy a birthday cake on or around the date of their egg retrievals and either keep some of the cake in the freezer or buy a new cake each year and celebrate it as a type of birthday.

I do believe that when things are out of sight, they are out of mind. The challenge in the Always Connected ritual is to keep the energy light and positive, and to continuously celebrate the beauty of life as present in these frozen eggs. For many people, there is a great personal judgment, often reinforced through medicine, about the quantity and quality of eggs that are retrieved. I try to remind my patients that a party can be any size and that sometimes the best parties are the smallest. When you hold a space to proudly commemorate the retrieval of your eggs, you are energetically connected to those pieces of you, no matter the distance, location, or time.

## TIMING, NOT TIME

"Am I too old to have a baby?" I have been asked this question thousands of times. When I was in my earlier years of medical practice, I tended to follow more traditional guidelines about age and fertility; since then, I have veered far from these standards. "It depends. I think that timing is more important than time," is how I now almost always respond.

After seeing people try unsuccessfully to conceive during a set period that seemed perfect for their reproductive clock, I've come to realize that even if it's the "right time," it still might not happen. In this book, we've explored some of the reasons conception does not take place, even if your ovaries are relatively young. But there is another more mysterious element that can contribute to the cosmic timing of your conception and pregnancy. It has to do with the greater timing in the story of your life's unfolding.

It can be frustrating to feel ready to have children while waiting for all the pieces to come together. I sometimes see my clients pushing hard against what I call the flow of the universe, and sometimes this push leads them into more and more Western medical intervention. While this can override our own biology to produce pregnancy, it can also be impacted by unseen and unknown forces.

Even if laboratory results, ultrasounds, and retrieval numbers look great, people can still fall into an unexplained infertility category. When this happens, I often ask what can be learned by stepping back and considering the greater picture of a client's life. Sometimes the events that need to take place in the future are dependent upon an exact infrastructure from the past; that is, events have to occur a particular way in the past for the future to happen the way the universe intends it to. But this is very difficult to determine, even in the energetic realm.

One of the hardest things to face as a potential parent is if—even if you are ready—your child's spirit might not be. Stepping back to trust in the great unknown is exceedingly difficult, particularly when your culture suggests that every day you wait, you are less and less likely to have that child.

Sacha was 42 when she came to see me. Her first question was if I intuitively thought she could conceive. She had been married years ago but had never wanted to have a child with her ex and was currently single. She would be a single mom by choice.

"Do you think you can?" I answered back.

She confidently responded, "I *know* I can, but my doctors are all discouraging me and I'm beginning to be afraid that I can't. Everyone tells me how hard single parenthood is." She shared how everyone in her life—doctors, friends, and family—told her she was too old to have a baby, and that it was tough to be a single mother. Because she was African American and grew up in Harlem, there was also a lot of trauma associated with being a single mom in her community and in her own family.

I reminded her that she had power over the narrative and opinions she allowed into her energy, and if she felt healthy and ready, she should have faith in that. I also helped her to connect to the spirit of her child through meditation, and at the end of our session we both felt a strong and very bright energy that wanted to come in. I closed by telling her I believed in her and that I didn't need to see her again.

Two-and-a-half years later, Sacha called me to set up an appointment. The following Tuesday morning, just as I was asking God to show me a sign of encouragement that my work was in alignment with God's intent for me, Sacha showed up for her appointment—on the wrong day, at the wrong time. She informed me that she had become pregnant after just one try, which happened the month after our session. She had used a donor's sperm and conceived via nonmedicated intrauterine insemination (IUI).

She said, "Dr. Von, you were the only person who believed in my body's health and my vision of motherhood. Your encouragement helped me to finally believe that I could become pregnant. You will always have a special place in my heart and in my son's life."

She added that after her child was born, she met the love of her life and that they were getting married and had discussed having more children. Sacha trusted in a very unconventional path toward motherhood. Throughout her journey, she had to conquer many fears about timing, being a single parent, and her age, but ultimately, her connection to her child's spirit outweighed the fears. She trusted in a different sort of timing. She trusted that she could be loved by a partner after motherhood, and she listened when the energetic whisper—or in this case, the shout—of her fierce little boy said, "I am ready for you, mama."

## UNSTRUCTURED TIME AND FERTILITY

Think back to the "empty" moments of childhood when you had ample time to dream and imagine. Can you remember the capacity that you had to create out of the emptiness? When is the last time you experienced a day, or even an hour, that was not filled with media, exercise, commuting, or a specific task-oriented achievement? The tie between empty, unstructured time and imagination is strong—so much so that when we over-determine our schedule and experiences, we disconnect from the part of our being that dreams and creates.

There are downfalls to living in a capitalist economy based on production and consumption. Capitalism relies on the commodification of eating, dressing, exercising, and even spending time with friends and family. For many of us, our identity is often tied to our output, production, and success. This can be sustainable for some, but there is also a danger that certain core aspects of self can be lost, ignored, and undernourished when the emphasis is placed solely on what you are *doing* versus how you are *being*. Your value as a human being is not measured by your productivity or how much you do. Unfortunately, it is much harder than any other time in our planet's history to practice being versus doing.

Why is unstructured time to simply be so essential to fertility? Engagement in the world requires engagement of your nervous system. Stress hormones (such as adrenaline) work on negative feedback systems, meaning your body produces biochemicals on demand. Like any system that works on demand, it can break or grow overused and tired. The effects of constant "doing" without sufficient "not doing" creates a society that does not take time to reflect on the adverse effects of constant productivity.

If we don't provide time to think about the effects of our collective actions, how do we know that our actions are even effective or meaningful? And how do we provide enough unstructured time to dream and imagine better and more unified ways of being human and new pathways for stewardship of the Earth for our children? A simple yet powerful practice for learning to trust in cosmic timing comes with the ritual of meditation.

A brief disclaimer: I must confess that I am a chronic over-doer. I left home early and have made my way in the world as a self-employed doctor and healer. A few years ago, I found myself at the end of a great cycle. I had lived and manifested the dream I'd created in my early 20s, but I had no free time or extra space to tap in and dream up my next evolution. I was overscheduled, tired, and stressed. I decided to do something radical, which for me meant returning to my roots. I traded all of my fitness classes for restorative yoga and meditation, and I kept blank holes in my schedule. I journaled about the ways I was being present in the now, and connected deeply with the powerful seven-year-old manifestor within.

To my surprise, the essence of my being was not hard to access. The simple act of providing space and emptiness allowed my soul's mission to shine through. I realized somewhere along the way that I had associated "being" with anxiety and fear. I felt that to be successful, I constantly needed to be planning and strategizing. Production and action felt safe; somehow, "doing" protected me and kept me viable in the world.

It was then that I understood how much of our value as humans we associate with our success and productivity. Without time to reflect, we repeat the same situations again and again. When we don't have time to ourselves, without hyperstimulation, we forget how to trust ourselves. We forget how to tap into our unconscious, which is teeming with messages that cannot reach us if we are overly focused on productivity. When we blindly trust a map, we sometimes cover unnecessary distance and forget to take in the environment along the way. But the map is not the territory, and timing is more important than time.

## Spiritual Fertility Essentials

In this chapter, you learned that cosmic timing is the most important type of time. Fertility is often chalked up to the "ticking" biological clock; however, when you use the tools of intuition, your relationship to time often changes. Observing life through the practice of your intuition helps restore your belief in your own ability to heal and understand the messages of your body.

The modern emphasis on individualism has given us many gifts, but the trade-off has been a break in the comfort and *knowing* that the tribe and collective once provided. Fertility is both an individual act and an act for the collective. And the choice to have a child is one of the biggest you will ever make. Fear is a prominent emotion that accompanies conception, pregnancy, birth, and parenthood. But the remedy for fear is finding the magic in your life through observing symbols, synchronicity, and cosmic timing. Practicing this not only changes the way you perceive reality; it also impacts the way reality unfolds around you. This, in turn, balances your nervous system and your hormones, creating a more stable and supportive environment for conception.

# Chapter 8

# How Our Ancestors and Spirit Guides Aid in the Fertility Journey

Many energy doctors and shamans share the belief that we are influenced by the ones who preceded us. Just like relationships in life, some of these ancestral connections are stronger than others. They sometimes have a particular interest in a genealogy continuing, although this is not always the case. It is not uncommon for a member of a family to pass away close to the time of a new member being born. Often, these two energies meet in the entry/exit to Earth. This encounter creates an eternal relationship, forming a karmic circle that, similar to a prayer circle, connects and supports that child energetically.

In Chapter 2, we explored ways to identify the impacts of transgenerational trauma on your fertility. Perhaps in that time of reflection, you also discovered the positive influences from your past. Identifying the ancestors with whom you resonate is a powerful foundational step in finding your energetic guides.

Guides are both real and symbolic, and provide energetic counsel and leadership. They are the avatars and expression of the most important aspects of you: your spirit and your life purpose. Certain friends also share a kinship and energetic resonance with us. They, too, serve as guides when we are in crisis or need. Events, especially intense events, bind us together. Much of what we value in our friends and family is their loyalty and partnership in navigating difficult times, as they are occurring and looking back later. Guides provide the same type of loyalty and partnership.

These karmic connections can be carried down through generations, particularly in more traditional cultures, where marriage was often orchestrated to strengthen the bonds of community. Entire religions, like Hinduism and Confucianism, were built around cataloguing and revering karmic connections.

You can also use karmic circles to more deeply understand the major themes of your most resonant connections. Dear friends from childhood with whom you have remained in contact might have entirely different lives and paths, and yet the same things that connected and bound you as children will often be present and apparent in your later years.

Here are some suggestions for creating a map that will help you to identify the karmic connections in your life:

- Look for relatives who passed away shortly before your conception or birth, because you passed these ancestors in the cosmic hallway as you entered Earth.

- Observe the signs of nature—in particular, your spirit animals and animals that hold a special resonance for you.

- Identify how you were named, and whom you were named after, because often you will share resonance with that ancestor.

- Explore your family lineage using the tools of intuition. Sit down with your family tree, and circle the ancestors you feel intuitively drawn toward, even if you know nothing about them.

- Reconnect with imaginary friends and visions from your childhood. These avatars can provide information about your spirit guides. Children's imaginations are open and fluid, and not yet governed by the rational mind.

- Stay open to different concepts and energies, even if they sound abstract and unproven.

The first and often most difficult step in identifying your divine guidance is trusting your intuition enough to let go of the need to rationally understand messages you might be receiving from the universe and from your guides.

When my client Amy called me for a scheduled consultation, her first words were, "Something led me to you and I just feel we were meant to work together." She went on to explain that although she had set up this consult months ago, just the week prior her father had handed her a business card. He had recently met an old friend from his company in Vietnam, someone he had not seen in over 40 years. When Amy's father shared with his old friend his daughter's difficulties with infertility, the man responded that his daughter was a fertility doctor, and pulled a business card out of his wallet, suggesting the two connect.

These two men had survived a vicious war. They fought together and protected each other. Fifty years later, hundreds of miles away from each other, the card that Amy's father placed in her hand was mine—given to him by my father.

"We were meant to work together," she said again. Our fathers had confirmed what she had already been guided toward. When Amy walked into my office for our meeting, I was somewhat taken aback. Her eyes and smile somehow were similar to mine. We looked as if we could be cousins. I felt the importance of acknowledging our connection while also beginning to investigate why Amy was not conceiving.

We began our session with a small prayer of gratitude to our fathers and the ancestral spirits that had kept them both safe. It was a deeply touching moment for both of us, which Amy would later reflect back on as being very important on her path to conception. Reconnecting to prayer was an essential step in her healing.

### THE GUIDES OF EARTH AND SKY

I have repeatedly witnessed the powerful healing that can take place when you ask for support from your ancestral line, particularly in reproduction. Of course, guides can be found in many forms in addition to those of your ancestors. I learned as a child that God dwelled in all things. I made sense of the concept of the Holy Spirit, one of the three branches of the divinity in Christianity, by imagining that the Holy Spirit worked through humans, animals, and nature to express the messages that God was sending us. In this way, I perceived the energy of the cosmos all around me, especially infusing animals and nature. At times, it felt like I could hear the messages that they each expressed—and I would often turn to the trees, flowers, birds, and sky for comfort, particularly when I was lonely, in pain, and confused.

When I later studied Shintoism and Eastern religions, I discovered that other cultures throughout time also believed that even the smallest of organic and inorganic life on our planet contained the essence of the Divine. In Shintoism, a boulder molded and caressed by time, wind, and water could contain a wise and patient ancient spirit. A similar philosophy has long been at work in North America through the belief and spiritual stewardship of indigenous people. Respect for Mother Earth and Father Sky, as well as all the cycles of life and death on Earth, is crucial to a spiritual practice that believes a binding and eternal energy is at the center of all things.

These days, people seldom look to the guides of Earth and sky for support. We have forgotten that sometimes the best way to answer a question is to ask a tree, a river, a mountain, or a star. Human beings are secretly ashamed, sad, and guilty for the harm that has befallen Earth, and in response we avoid contact with Earth and her messengers. But when all around you is infused with God, then all around you can serve as a guide.

## DRAFTING YOUR UPSTAIRS TEAM

Sometimes we literally need someone to give us permission: permission to act radically, to change our path, to trust in a vision or idea, or to take the time and nourishment needed for healing. Often, the less we trust ourselves, the more we look to others to determine our path. While people in our lives can help in this way, it is truly hard for them to do so without interpreting our needs through their own needs and fears. It has become harder than ever to find people who can simply listen without this filter. A guide is meant to help you along the path, to show you a way, but it is ultimately you who must decide to take it. And, of course, it is you who must also do the walking.

Alice contacted me after five years of trying to conceive. She mapped out a history of unexplained infertility, which was diagnosed at age 34 after three failed IUI cycles and two failed IVF rounds. Now aged 37, she wanted to come to peace with not being a mother. She and I worked to identify the possible blocks that might be getting in the way of pregnancy, but every step of the way, I found that Alice was free of the more likely causes of infertility.

She had not experienced insurmountable trauma in this lifetime, and her relationship to the universe, her family, and her partner were all healthy and supportive. She herself was a well-known holistic healer and herbalist who had a powerful spiritual practice that she developed and supported in the painful times of infertility. Her day-to-day work helped make a difference in the lives of others, and she was passionate and content in her life's purpose.

"You need an energetic advisory board," were the first words I said to Alice.

"What's that?" she responded.

"It's your hand-selected energy advisers, so to speak, made up of ancestors, your guides here on Earth, and the energetic forces of the universe that have an interest in your destiny."

Alice was at a critical moment on her path. She was feeling pressured either to use a donor egg or to adopt, but she was overwhelmed and confused as to whether either was right for her. "I used to be certain that I didn't want to conceive using another woman's egg—it just never felt right for me—but am I making a mistake?"

Alice had begun to second-guess herself, a common pattern in the fertility journey. Self-doubt can feel like an evil virus in your body, sabotaging everything positive and forward-moving in your life. However, self-doubt has one or two positive qualities. To begin with, feeling doubt means that you are free. The movement and awareness of different emotional and intellectual states—and the free will to sit in one longer than the other, even if it is critical and negative—defines a mind that is expansive and intelligent.

It can be difficult to come to peace with the decision to stop trying to conceive. The current narrative encourages people to continue to try no matter what, to never give up hope, and to persist through infertility like a warrior. Alice wanted to stop the fight but needed support and confirmation that it was okay to do so. As her friends, family, and medical team continued to encourage her to keep trying to conceive or to adopt, the reality was she wanted to stop but felt that she couldn't say so. In times like these, when you need to turn doubt into assurance and action but have little to no support from your community, you can look to your guides for assistance. Alice needed support from her higher self, not the world.

We set out to connect with and establish her energetic council. I first led Alice through a ritual that I call Council of Emotions (see sidebar on page 154), a meditation that clarifies the dominant emotions influencing the situation at hand. Many cultures have a practice of a council of elders who could be consulted for wisdom when the tribe was at a crossroads. In my expansion of this ritual, I suggested Alice envision the people who might embody her council of emotions. I had her name, draw, and describe in detail what each council member looked and felt like. She drafted a team of six, two of whom she described as being her head ancestral guides, who had been with her throughout her life. She began to honor each of their memories with simple rituals of acknowledgment, like an offering of fruit or incense. And each time Alice felt overwhelmed and confused as to how she should proceed with her fertility, she would talk to her council for advice.

I asked Alice to start the practice of automatic writing as she talked to her guides. Automatic writing involves stream-of-consciousness writing that uses free association rather than rational thought; it's a common magical practice and a way to commune with and receive guidance from our higher self and guides, while bypassing the part of the mind that might wish to control our narrative. Automatic writing can also be used to express your unconscious thoughts and emotions, serving as a conduit by which vital messages can be delivered to you.

One morning, Alice's scheduled call was delayed by a bad storm that knocked out power in her hometown. We rescheduled for the following day. The next morning, Alice called with a very calm and centered energy. I felt that something had dramatically shifted in her being. She went on to explain that she had received "a clear message from Grandmother energy."

Grandmother and Grandfather energy are terms that describe deeply loving and supportive ancestral energy; some tribal practices acquaint these forces with the eternal masculine and feminine energies of the cosmos.

"I was sitting in my bedroom early yesterday morning, listening to the rain and doing the automatic writing process that you suggested," she explained. "I just lit a candle when I felt moved to ask my great-great-grandmother to show me a sign as to what I should do. I told her that whatever she said was how I would proceed, and that I would put my full faith and trust in her council."

Alice's great-great-grandmother was one of the two major guides she had previously identified. "I began to write over and over again the sentence, 'Let it go and it will happen by the light of the waning crescent moon. Let it go and it will happen by the light of the waning crescent moon.' And at that exact moment, the power went out from the storm. But I had already lit the candle, so even though all else around me was dark, I could still see the words."

I worked with Alice for another two sessions until her trust, belief, and boundaries were fully established and secure. She was no longer subject to other people's opinions about her fertility. I concluded our work by writing in an e-mail, "When you have the protection of the cosmic grandmothers on your team, you have personal access to the wisdom and security of the universe. It's like being able to use the backdoor of the universal temple, the door that leads directly to the kitchen table where your grandmother sits, while many others have to wait for someone to answer the doorbell."

The message, *Let it go and it will happen by the light of the waning crescent moon,* comforted Alice and gave her permission to let go of extensive fertility treatments. It might not have made sense to anyone else—but for Alice, it was radical. My work with her was always specifically about getting out of the way of her access and belief in her own intuition and desire. While there were several times when she looked to me for confirmation that there was a baby spirit connected to her, from the beginning I decided not to share the energetic information I perceived about her future children. It would not have helped her healing process. The injury that occurred to Alice through failed fertility treatments was an injury to her relationship to self and to the universe. Had I filled the role of guide, Alice would never have been given the opportunity to remember that she herself had this divine access, and that she had only forgotten how to trust in it and in her higher self.

Alice wrote a powerful letter to her friends and family explaining she no longer wanted anyone's advice on her fertility. She acknowledged she had needed their support and advice before, and that she was grateful for all the time, love, and financial support they had provided—but that the issue of her fertility was no longer to be discussed. There was some pushback, but for Alice the sovereign act of pulling back all of the energetic cords that she had woven as a result of self-doubt and fear was the final step in healing.

Years passed and I sometimes meditated on Alice, as I do with all the gorgeous souls I have worked with over the years. I remembered the automatic writing quote that she had found so much comfort in and wondered what her grandmother guide had meant by it. I often experience through the energetic fabric of the universe the synchronicity of thinking about a client and then being contacted by them, even after many years have passed. So I was pleasantly not surprised to receive an e-mail from Alice the next week.

"Seven years have passed," she wrote, "and I can't tell you how much our work together changed everything for me. I had not realized, back then, how much of my power I had given away. I stopped trying, didn't adopt, focused on life and love . . . but I wanted to tell you that I finally understand the message. I'm eight months pregnant."

I began to sob as I understood the beauty and wisdom of what her guides had told her. The end of the menstrual cycle can be as erratic as when it began in adolescence— and often, the two reflect each other. Cycles that start off irregular, heavy, and long will oftentimes end the same way. I look to menarche, or the onset of the menstrual cycle, when I work with perimenopause. Specifically, the hormones LH and FSH fluctuate in relation to estrogen; sometimes, this fluctuation will strongly stimulate ovulation, even as the systems are beginning to shut down. Alice had entered these waning years of her moon cycle at age 45, and her body—which had not responded to reproductive medicine—surprised her with the perfect storm of hormonal catalyst and the opportunity to conceive.

Of course, Alice had to trust in her intuition and guides, and there was no guarantee that simply letting go would result in future fertility, but the healing and return to self that happened along the way was worth the sacrifice of certainty. A few months later, I received a baby announcement from Alice. Her daughter was a redheaded beauty, who, as Alice explained in the card, was named after her great-great-grandmother.

## Exercise: *Council of Emotions*

Many cultures have a practice of consulting with a council of elders for wisdom when the tribe is at a crossroads. To help you connect with your ancestors and energetic guides, I suggest that you imagine gathering your emotions around a symbolic fire. Let each emotion have a place of equality. Speak first from the emotion that feels most comfortable, while taking note of how much time you allot for this emotion to express itself, as well as how your body feels and looks as you visualize.

Now, make your way around the council of emotions, providing equal space and time for each aspect to express itself. Pay particular attention to the emotions that you would prefer to skip or the ones that get interrupted by your more dominant and comfortable "attendees." You can expand the exercise to envision the people who might embody this council of emotions. Create avatars for each emotion. Be specific by giving them names, and draw and describe in detail what each council member looks and feels like.

### YOUR GUIDES ALWAYS PICK UP

As children, we are all magical manifestors capable of spinning imagination into reality through games, art, and play. I often feel that we discredit the wisdom and intelligence of children, most likely in an effort to protect them from our fears and traumas. Children are very open channels, and they are capable of accessing their spirit guides very easily.

Imaginary friends are often spirit guides that fill the energetic roles of protectors and playmates during important periods of spiritual and mental development. The most powerful and soul-connected of your guides are the imaginary friends who are with you in this lifetime and beyond. They never leave your side, and even if you haven't spoken in ages, they will always, *always* pick up the phone when you reach out.

After the birth of my daughter, I experienced what I now describe as a spiritual civil war. Raising a small child in New York City is physically and emotionally demanding, and because my work also includes the psychic and physical care of my patients, I was left with little in my own personal reserves, despite my best self-care efforts. What I had done before to care for myself, including how I had exercised and nourished myself with food and the psychological and spiritual tools I had cultivated, no longer worked. The transition to becoming a mother had forced me, as it does all new parents, into an identity crisis. All of the armor that I had built during my earlier life to defend my sensitive soul was no longer of any use. I was flooded by waves and waves of psychic and energetic information, and there were times when I could not differentiate between what was mine and what was someone else's. I felt ungrounded and unsure of myself.

One of the first questions I learned to ask as a practicing intuitive was if what I was feeling was mine, or if it was someone else's. During this time, I could not tell the two apart. Few people speak of how the first few years of a child's life are some of the most difficult for an empathic parent. As an empath, you are often extremely aware of the needs of the other—and a child is the greatest representation of the other. To this day, I bow down to my daughter for teaching me, finally, what it means to construct the boundaries of self. The beauty is that in this vulnerable period, you can realign with your soul purpose, as well as the radiant truth of what it is to be alive. But you can just as easily be frayed and exhausted by the face-to-face conversations that occur: namely, between you, God, and the meaning of being alive.

It was during this period of personal reconstruction, after my spiritual civil war, that I returned to a practice of connecting with and trusting my guides. I had forgotten to ask for support. But I learned that I could return to the guides I had found in childhood—the angels and healing forces of light—as well as those I met during my travels and studies with shamans in the American Southwest. I had ignored an entire team of guidance.

As a young child, I attended a church camp in the mountains of New Mexico. During a family outing to Santa Fe, I wandered into a store that sold magical figures from world religions, as well as the spiritual tools of local tribe members. I was in awe of the magical devices and powerful symbols, and although I had been taught to distrust and not participate in this type of "occult" material, I felt completely at home and alive. I picked out a small silver pendant of a bear with what looked like a bolt of lightning carved into it. The clerk explained to me that this was a medicine bear made by a local Navajo jeweler, and that it granted healing powers to whomever wore it. He said bears were great healers and symbols of strength because they continue to fight even after they have been hurt. My sister Jenny helped me pay for it, and we left the store to find my family. My older brother Jim had also purchased something at the store, a statue of a Hindu god. My parents were so angry at him for buying an idol of an unknown deity, which they would later make him throw away into the forest, that they didn't notice the bear medicine around my neck. Later, when they asked me where it came from, I lied and said it was from the church gift shop.

Years later I asked my brother about this event, and he told me that he had secretly pocketed the small statue and only pretended to throw it away. I laughed, thinking about how he and I were certainly from the same "clan." To this day, I wear bear medicine protection and honor the spirit and signs of its energy. I have also had several run-ins with bears over the years, but none as powerful as my first.

Just as we look to ancestral guides to show us the way, we can also look to the animal and plant spirits of Earth to be our guides. I have had many encounters with animals that I consider to be important events in my own healing. On the drive years ago, when I first recognized and connected to the spirit of my daughter in the West Texas desert, I also discovered one of my personal animal spirits: the raven. On a long hike alone through Big Bend National Park, I sat down to rest next to a *tinaja*, a type of watering hole in the desert. Tinajas tend to be very sacred sites because they provide the substance of life, water, in an otherwise harsh environment. They are often also burial grounds for animals that fall in and, unable to climb out, die. It was at this tinaja that I first noticed the call of the raven.

"You are a beautiful soul," I said out loud as I snapped a photograph. Something in that moment helped me to feel supported and loved by the universe and the earth. In indigenous spirituality, the raven represents the power of magic, mysticism, and healing. It seemed that it had purposely signed on to watch my back that day. I am almost always in proximity to ravens, so much so that I have grown to take it for granted that wherever I am, ravens will also be there. I have always kept the photo of my first contact with Raven on my altar and still call on this guide to help me in my healing work.

You don't have to be in direct contact with animals to have them on your team, but often, once you do, they will manifest in your life, whether literally or symbolically. Guides play an important role in keeping you on your spiritual path. Imagine the old cartoon depiction of an angel and a devil sitting on opposite shoulders, debating what to do next. Guides serve such a purpose in our lives, directing us to the path that our higher self must take. They have the power to step in and push you back on track. Such was true for me.

In my early 20s, I was second-guessing my path as a healer. I already knew that I wanted to become a holistic doctor, but I was terrified and besieged by self-doubt. I had the map in my hand but was afraid to take the first steps: moving away from socially accepted Western medicine to the more obscure path of alternative medicine. I had learned from a shaman at age 17 that when overcome with self-doubt, a journey alone to the wilderness will set the stage for you to find clarity and confidence. So I packed up my camping gear and drove west. About halfway through the six-hour drive, I began to feel feverish. By the time I got to the national park and set up camp, I was fully in the throes of a violent and intense flu.

The best I could do was boil water for tea and wrap myself tightly in extra clothing to warm my shaking body. It was nighttime by then, and I decided to sleep there because the nearest town was more than an hour away and the park store was closed. "I wish I knew a medicine that could be used to heal in situations like these," I said to myself. "There must be something else to do or take besides prescriptions from the grocery store."

Of course, I had already found the answer to this question in the brilliance of acupuncture and holistic medicine, but for the first time, I understood its true necessity. The fever grew and grew, and the cold desert floor seeped into my tent and sleeping bag. In my delirium, I brought my tea and a bottle of honey, my only medicine to soothe my symptoms, into my tent, a dangerous thing to do when camping in the wild. After tossing and turning for hours, I fell asleep, only to awaken in the dead of night to the sound of a large animal rooting around my campsite. I knew instantly that it was a bear.

Realizing my mistake in bringing the honey inside, I froze in fear as I heard the muffled sound of the bear's breath at my tent door. I could have sat up, turned on the lights, and made noise to scare it away—but I was weak and exhausted from fever . . . so I prayed instead. I told the bear how much I appreciated the visit and how thankful I was that he was watching over me. I asked him to let me rest and to leave my site so I could heal. "If you can do this, I'll never question my path as a healer again."

After several more minutes, the bear disappeared, and while I remained terrified, I heard its message and committed to my path. Once dawn broke, I zipped open my tent to find the site totally wrecked. My camp stove was on the ground and my kitchen utensils were spread around everywhere. A ranger came by to say that a bear had been reported last night.

"I know," I said. Although still very unwell, I stayed another day to sleep and recover. I drove back to Austin, Texas, that Sunday and without hesitation woke up on Monday morning, drove to the AOMA at Austin's Graduate

School of Integrative Medicine, filled out an application, and paid the deposit.

Bear medicine is strong medicine—it does not mess around.

Our fears can keep us from taking the next steps along our path, but as my brilliant husband says, "You can't outrun your destiny."

## SPIRIT GUIDES AND YOUR BABY

Your guides are powerful ambassadors of your citizenship as a spiritual being. It is miraculous to consider all of the events of the past that contributed to each of us being born. A grand orchestration of people, places, and timing all had to fall into place for you to be conceived. Each ancestor, and their struggle to live out their destiny, is embodied in you. Each element that it takes to make up life on Earth can be found in your body.

I have yet to work with a person who did not have any guides, but many people are afraid to connect and speak to theirs. Zoe set up a session to get more clarity on whether she should have a child. She felt that many factors were keeping her from finding love and starting a family, but she longed for both. Something had injured Zoe's original connection to the universe. I could sense her distrust and skepticism, even through her sincere desire to heal and have a child.

Zoe recalled a memory of being conceived with a twin that died in utero. She told me that she felt a part of her melancholy came from never having healed from the loss of this original sibling. "Perhaps that is who you are longing for now," I said. "Maybe that is the spirit that is knocking on your door. I want you to close your eyes and ask this spirit a question. Any question will do, like how is the weather, even."

Zoe's energy shifted, and she began to cry hysterically. While she felt 100 percent comfortable with my contacting and communicating with the spirit of her child, she herself felt blocked and unable to do the same. After several minutes of gut-wrenching sobs, she began to gather herself and speak. "I have so much belief in spirit and God, but I don't feel worthy or capable of direct communication."

Zoe's grandmother, who had raised her, had recently passed away, so I asked Zoe to start a journal of letters to her grandmother, as well as to the spirit of her child/children. The exercise would safely open the lines of communication and allow Zoe to connect and ask questions independently. I also mentioned that her grandmother would now help her spirit baby to find his way to Earth.

When you hear the whisper of a child's spirit and are struck by the desire to become a parent, it is easy to forget the influence that your child's energy is already having on your life. Each child brings a new karma to a family, and the effects of this karma begin before conception. I have seen mountains moved to get two people into the same room to meet and fall in love, in order for a child to be born. When you recognize and communicate with your guides, you display your trust and faith in your child's spirit and intent to be born. You also open up direct lines of communication for calling your baby home.

## Exercise: *Letters to Your Unborn Child*

Sometimes, one of the easiest ways to connect to your upstairs team and to your future children is to simply write them a letter. I suggest creating a template within a journal or writing e-mails to these spirits. Some of my patients have even created e-mail addresses for their future children and started to write them messages long before they were even conceived. It is a powerful practice of faith, and more often than not brings many emotions to the surface because of its direct nature.

"But what am I supposed to say?" is a question I often hear. Here is a list of topics that have proven to be both powerful and healing:

- The love story of how you and your partner met

- Memories from childhood of your grandparents and ancestors

- What you like to do on a fun weekend or on vacation (baby spirits really like this one)

- Stories about your family pets or animals that you grew up with or currently have

- Details of what inspires you, such as the music, books, and movies you like, and why

- Descriptions of what a normal day of your life looks like and how you would share that day with them

This exercise is one of the most difficult in this book because it brings you face-to-face with any unconscious blocks or fears that might be keeping you from believing you will conceive and have a child. There is an ancient Chinese medicine saying: "The song that cannot be sung out from the heart must be a very sad song, indeed."

Essentially, the hardest thoughts and emotions to express are the ones we keep closest and most guarded. Beginning the practice of corresponding with the energy of a lost ancestor or a future child will present you with a literal path of expression to those who are most capable of holding space and loving you unconditionally. Remember, there is no shame in asking for help. Begin to set the model that you want your child to live by, even long before your newborn arrives in your arms.

## Spiritual Fertility Essentials

In this chapter, we started to incorporate the work of the prior chapters into a practical system for you to use. The goal of spiritual fertility is to empower you to connect with your intuition and to become its advocate, as well as the advocate of your child's spirit. Listening and practicing from your intuition can be challenging, and there will be times when you doubt your ability to interpret messages from the universe. There will also be times when you are simply too afraid of a potential answer that you fear even asking the question.

We also spoke about how to set aside the opinions of others—in particular, the ones who are closest and most influential—in exchange for your own wisdom and knowledge. The universe and cosmic timing are on your side, and they show their support to you daily through symbols and synchronicities. When you fall into doubt about your fertility, you need not look far for support. It will be there for you to discover, infused into the day-to-day magic of your life.

# Chapter 9

# Karmic Connections, Spirit Contracts, and Past Lives

In the beginning of this book, I described the sacred moment when I became aware of my daughter's energy in my own field. The energetic exchange that she and I had at that moment, however subtle, confirmed an agreement that we both went on to fulfill: I was to be her mother in this lifetime, and she was to be my child.

Around the time of this agreement, as I explored realms of thought and consciousness at the university I attended, a friend mentioned to me the theory that we have karmic relationships with the significant players of our lives. That is, in a past life, our mothers might have been our sisters, our fathers might have been our sons, as well as many other possible combinations when it comes to the people we know and with whom we are intimately familiar. The thought, however fascinating, seemed complex and impossible at the time. However much I had fallen away from my Christian roots, I still held the notion that our eternal souls, although they lived on in heaven, did not pass back to this side of consciousness. I had, like many others, felt a sense of connection and deep familiarity with certain people, and this seemed to suggest an energetic history. But part of me felt that acknowledging this karma didn't really change anything. Having these connections was sufficient without having to name or identify their origin or relationship.

But as I gained worldly experience and suffered the mistakes and heartbreaks and courageous carelessness that often occur in one's late teens, I gained a new understanding of the key role of these karmic players. Many of those incipient experiences came with the liberation I discovered being free from my parents' rule and finally being allowed to be my own individual.

I am the last of three children, and my sister and brother were more than ten years older than me when I was born. As a child, I often asked my mother why she chose to have me so long after the others. She would always reply, "God told me to have another child." This was lovely to hear at a young age (it feels good to be chosen by God, after all), but it also placed an extremely heavy burden on me to be an example of godliness. I was the perfect child; other than my debilitating asthma, I expressed love and compassion for all beings and was kind to all others at school, church, and home. My sensitive soul took the messages of Christ to heart, and I sacrificed my own individual needs for those who were in more need than I was.

All of this changed when I was 15 and I felt the cruel sting of hypocrisy from my church community by way of judgment for the simple act of dyeing my hair purple. Something in me snapped awake. It was devastating to realize that those around me didn't practice the compassion and nonjudgment I had learned as cornerstones of the Christian way of life. I have always felt that the karmic contract I made with my parents was as much about fostering a deep spirituality as it was about setting up a system for me to rebel against.

Having a system to rebel against set me on my path of exploring alternative consciousness, spirituality, and health. Something in my soul revolts any time it senses injustice in how one individual is treated differently and cruelly, compared to the rest of the group. This early sense of advocating for the individual led to my work in women's health and fertility. There were times in that massive period of rebellion and exploration when I suffered greatly and came face-to-face with the depths of my soul, barely retrieving it on my way to the next life lesson. I lived with thirst and courage. I traveled alone, camping with bears in the wilderness, rock climbing with a renegade group of anarchist lost boys, studying with shamans, driving 24 hours straight to the Pacific Ocean for no other reason than to see the full moon on the water, living with an older man who was preparing for the end of the world at the millennium, and reading everything I could get my hands on. Looking back, it feels like I practically fit 20 years of living into the years between ages 17 and 21.

In 2000, when the world in fact did not end, I decided that I wanted to be in it instead of on its outskirts. But I was lost and tired. I needed a banner in the crowd. How could I find my path to service when I had so many fundamental problems with the normative systems of society? Medicine called me back. The Hippocratic oath was fair and equal to all, at least in theory, and I knew that my gift of healing could be useful there. Working from the guidance of spirit alone, I registered late for a premed lab class that was, much to my annoyance, held on a Saturday morning at 8 I arrived late and found the one open chair in the back.

Unbeknownst to me, I sat down next to one of those banner holders and key players of my life—a woman whom I have undeniably known for thousands of lives, my dearest friend in this lifetime, Heather Kim. Heather, like me, was a courageous lover of life—and she, too, was at a significant crossroads. We met there that day and were inseparable ever after. We each went on to become doctors and to serve and defend women and children from crushing systems that seek to oppress. I honestly am not sure if either of us could have alone successfully carried out the journey from that first lab class to our individual practices. I can say without doubt that we saved each other, and that our meeting was 100 percent planned and orchestrated before we were even born.

As children and young adults, we discuss a book after reading it. We explore key themes and characters as a way to learn at a deeper level. It's sometimes only after this discussion that we get the most significant message of the novel. Similarly, we can assume that there are certain people and events that are set to occur in our lives without giving much thought as to why. But the post-discussion and analysis can unveil to us precious life lessons and themes. A retrospective look can reveal to us what was present all along.

I used to think that wisdom was impossible not to obtain, that simply living granted a person knowledge. Now I understand that the wisest of those I have met are the ones who were able to craft meaningful stories and myths from the milestones and major events of their lives. And the children that they had—as well as the ones they lost in miscarriage, termination, or death—were each significant figures in their story. Some contracts, after all, are simply powerful enough by just existing, even if they are never acted upon.

### Exercise: *Who Are Your Key Holders?*

Many roads in our lives become available to walk only after we have met certain people. Identify the main players in your life thus far. Imagine they each hold a sacred key to help you unlock a very important door to your life's purpose. These people often show up during times of great transition. What do these key holders have in common, and what is different about each of them? The resonance they share is a clue to the type of energy you are calling in this lifetime. Often, this energy will be reflected in the spirit of your child, as well. Your child is another important key holder along your path.

## KARMIC RELATIONSHIPS THAT TRANSCEND TIME

Some of my greatest heroes are my patients. I have sat with people in the most devastating spaces that a human can experience and have seen firsthand how the human spirit can alchemize tragedy into wisdom. That is not to say that the experience of going through miscarriage, stillbirth, and loss of a child ever truly leaves you—nor does it make you stronger, as the old saying suggests. If anything, it makes you more raw and vulnerable to the experience of being alive, with all of its delicate tenuousness. The philosopher Saint Augustine wrote that the best of humanity is practiced in faith, hope, and love. These are also the core tools that I remind my patients to access when they feel despair. In practice, you can observe the energetic impact these principles have on fertility.

Deborah was referred to me by a colleague at Carriage House Birth Doulas. The last decade has seen an exciting increase in education around childbirth, and doulas have spearheaded much of it. They are also at the battlefront of women's reproductive health, and because of their positioning, doulas witness many traumas related to fertility firsthand. Doulas are often my favorite people in the room. In general, they have an extraordinary sense of service to others and the kindest hearts. Trust me when I say you want a doula on your team.

Deborah had a normal and healthy first pregnancy with manageable morning sickness and fatigue. All of her normally scheduled ultrasounds came back positive up until week 25 of her pregnancy, when her positive and upbeat ultrasound technician suddenly shifted into a serious and withdrawn state. Something had changed—and something was very wrong. Previously undetected irregularities had developed in the fetus. The pregnancy ended at 26 weeks. Upon later analysis, a very rare and not inheritable genetic variation was found to be the cause, which gave some comfort to Deborah but still didn't answer why she had lost the baby.

There is an inventory of questions that most people scroll through while trying to make sense of losing a pregnancy. It almost always begins with a deep self-critique and includes waves of shame and guilt at the sense of having done something wrong or being inadequate as a mother. Deborah came to see me as she began to heal her body after the loss. Although she was doing well on the outside, internally she was full of unresolved grief and fear. "How do I get over this?" she asked.

"You don't," I replied. "But you do find ways to understand why. However, in my experience, those explanations often don't come fast." I never try and take away the grief from my patients too quickly, nor do I tell them to just get back up and keep trying, as many doctors suggest. Again, it's been my experience that in Western medicine, a person's age plays a major role in the fear she feels around the pressure to get pregnant. I've seen many a client over the years start trying to conceive again, too soon after an unresolved loss, simply because they feel their biological clock is ticking. For many, even strong fertility treatments cannot override womb break. It can only be healed with time, and that is the commodity that most people feel they are running out of.

The loss of a child is never something to be rushed through. Not taking the time to adequately mourn can produce more trauma, not just for the mother but for her future children, as well. The weight of being conceived to fix the heartbreak of a prior sibling's death is unfair to those who come after, and can lead to feelings of being loved conditionally and not solely for who they are. The wisdom of the heart and its connection to the uterus will only allow a subsequent pregnancy to occur once healing has taken place. And healing looks very different for everyone.

I encourage my clients to give themselves permission to feel all their feelings after a loss. Feeling is often the first thing they want to stop doing. Often, the daily reminders from the world—like e-mail notifications from baby apps and reminders of the Pinterest board they had created for the baby's room—are sufficient to catalyze a deep melancholy that is hard enough to navigate. Modern-day women hold in emotion. We censor ourselves to be more acceptable, to stick out less, and to avoid being perceived as overly emotional.

Over the years, many of my clients who have been through negative pregnancy tests, miscarriages, and loss have asked me how to manage the great sadness they feel. "Cry more," I tell them. "It helps release the energy from your body and prepare for the next pregnancy." Often, people still do not allow themselves to express their feelings fully, for fear of judgment—and of course, having to actually acknowledge their pain. Ultimately, it is as the great poet Robert Frost wrote: "The best way out is always through."

A miscarriage is a missed connection. And just like romantic love, there can be so much that is right about a potential life partner; they can be almost perfect, but loving someone is ultimately not enough of a reason to stay together. However, that doesn't mean there was no significance to the time you *did* spend together, however temporary. The karmic connections we encounter in life are there to help steer our paths and catalyze self-realization. Some practitioners in the realm of energy medicine describe miscarried children as transient spirits that are so pure of spirit that they cannot fully incarnate onto Earth. The closest thing they can experience to the physical realm is the womb. I have always liked this theory, and while it has resonated for a few of my clients over the years, it is ultimately too broad of an interpretation to be true for everyone. What I do suggest, and what applies to everyone I have worked with, is that the loss of a child is a significant event that requires examination, reflection, and time to heal. When we honestly take time to identify what felt right and what felt wrong, just as we would a romantic relationship, we often find answers that guide our path and that help to heal our womb break.

## THE UNINTENDED CONSEQUENCES
## OF THE SEXUAL REVOLUTION

The increase in infertility is one of the unintended consequences of the sexual revolution. In the 1970s, women began to disengage and silence their monthly connection to their uterus, either through oral contraceptives or detachment from menstrual bleeding, pain, and discomfort, in order to be able to gain economic status and to compete for jobs that had only been held by men.

The value that had once been placed on reproduction and being a mother was no longer sufficient. Women had to not only have and raise children, and do the bulk of the housework; they also had to get right back up and achieve the same success as their professional male counterparts. Although the freedom that developed during this time was essential for global economic growth, many of the exalted characteristics of the feminine prior to the sexual revolution gained negative connotations. Fast-forward to the modern-day economy; while there are more options for women to take maternity leave and preserve their fertility through egg freezing and reproductive medicine, the world still runs on an active, masculine-fueled ethic of overdoing and productivity.

I have met many women who simply don't know how to connect to their bodies, wombs, and reproductive cycles. They have been on oral contraceptives since college, and have been reassured that they are capable of doing everything that men do (plus get pregnant) as soon as they decide to. Women have been spoon-fed the notion that they can have everything—and they are exhausted and disconnected from their feminine essence as a result.

Countless times, I have asked women struggling to get pregnant how many hours a week they work, only to hear time and again that they are devoting an average of 60 hours a week to their job. Their sleep and sex drives suffer from so much doing. Quite simply, the expectations that society and modern women place on themselves and their reproductive systems are unreasonable.

A return to the feminine realm of intuition and connecting to the natural, internal rhythms of our bodies is not a return to a lesser form of intelligence—it's a return to a sense of balance that is desperately needed in our world, among both women and men.

This might be a good time to remind you that my roots are in feminism. Growing up, I fought against established patriarchy. The kind of oppression I experienced could have easily demolished my spirit instead of facilitating the growth of my gifts, as it did. Moreover, I am not suggesting that there is a veil that sharply separates masculine analytic thought from feminine intuitive wisdom. Both sides can freely cross over and participate—and many men are naturally gifted with a developed feminine, while many women are more comfortable in the realm of the masculine. It seems to me that the majority of people tend to stay on one side of the divide. The imbalance of energies is reflected in the way we as human beings live, love, and reproduce.

When I teach women receptivity and connecting to the womb in order to facilitate pregnancy, one of the first steps is learning to listen to their menstrual cycles. They often pull out apps, data for their tracked cycles, and basal body temperature charts they have turned into Excel sheets, which is all well and good. But the type of listening I am asking for requires a different kind of data collection. It is not linear; it seeks a direct and open line of communication between your uterus, your heart, and your mind. My father use to say, "There are only 13 inches between heaven and hell, and that is the distance between your heart and your head." To which I add the 16-inch descent from the heart to the uterus and the statement, "What you know in your uterus can be spoken through your heart."

Some seem to think that it is easy to act from intuition versus analysis, and that following your intuition is a lesser form of intelligence than analyzing all aspects of a situation through logic. Indeed, explaining your reason for doing something by simply saying "My intuition said it was the right thing to do" can sometimes come off as confusing and chaotic in a world that values explanation. However, once you have developed a methodical personal practice, you can trust in its validity and the messages that you receive.

Let's get back to the story of my client Deborah, whom I mentioned earlier in the chapter. She took the time needed to heal. Months went by, and although she was exceedingly busy with work and life, she made space to listen to her cycle and to grieve. She found ways to understand the significance in her life story of the loss of her first child, and came to the belief that the cosmic timing for that pregnancy was simply not correct.

Almost one year after the loss of her first child, she heard a small but clear whisper. "Hi," it said. It was the sound of her child's voice. It was different from the spirit she had felt and connected to before, but she immediately knew that it was, indeed, a hello meant for her. Naturally, she became pregnant the following cycle. Having walked through hell and back, she was now capable of sharing a deeper love than ever before, both for her unborn child and for herself.

## COMMUNICATING WITH YOUR SPIRIT BABY

Our greatest teachers are our partners and our children. They carry with them the blueprints for how to break into our most secure areas and take whatever they so desire. Carrie, a fertility coach herself, asked me if I had ever heard another baby spirit knocking at my door.

"Why do you ask?" I responded.

Carrie went on to describe the awareness of a baby spirit whom she felt had been with her for some time. "It's just not the right time," she said. "I've just raised my two boys, and I want to spend energy on my business of helping women."

"It's okay to tell her that, then," I said. "Just say with unconditional love and sovereignty that this isn't the right time, and allow her to make the choice to stick around or be free."

Carrie felt liberated. It had been hard for her to open up about her own desire to spend the energy that she had devoted to motherhood on herself and her career, especially because she was aware that the energy was coming from a potential daughter and she was curious after raising sons what it might be like to be the mother to a girl.

"In my belief system," I concluded, "energy and karmic connections are timeless—and if you don't meet in this lifetime, you can in another." Ultimately, the relationships that are absolutely necessary for our spiritual development are unavoidable. I share this affirmation with my clients, particularly when they are anxious or under the impression that everything and everyone that is intended for them will always find them.

Another hurdle faced when practicing receptive listening for the spirits of children is conquering the fear of hearing nothing. "What does it mean if I can't hear or feel my spirit baby?" is a question I am often asked. Some people are so afraid of not hearing someone speaking back that they hesitate to even try my meditations. For me, this typically indicates a need to go back to the earlier steps of identifying and clearing trauma that we spoke about in the first chapters of this book. Most of the time the blockages to connecting and communicating with a baby's spirit can be cleared, and the gentle presence of their spirit can be detected.

On occasion, I have encountered very shy and quiet baby spirits who prefer not to speak or make their presence too conspicuous. In these cases, I recommend holding a gentle and undemanding space for them to get comfortable in. After experiencing a safe and unconditionally loving space, these shy spirits always allow their presence to be known. Likewise, spirits can sometimes be exceedingly playful and mischievous, and will hide away from being known, as if it were a game of hide-and-seek. All I can say about these lovely souls is that they make the most feisty and energetic children and people!

## LOSS LEADS TO A NEW PATH

In the multiplex of our cosmic theater, we are all connected. Karmic connections and contracts that we make before incarnating into the world are real and often binding. I think back on the events of my lifetime (and the ones yet to happen) that had to occur to assist in my actualization. All of the events and people, both negative and positive, have catalyzed essential processes and reactions that have guided my path.

However painful and difficult to navigate, I have come to acknowledge, respect, and appreciate the failures and losses. The pressure to be perfect and to get everything right the first time is a self-imposed torture we submit to in order to avoid having to explore our fears and sadness. But not a single one of us, regardless of our economic status or nationality, will live an entire lifetime without experiencing loss, depression, sadness, and despair. However, only some will courageously risk having to experience all of the loss again, by choice, to follow the messages from their heart. Amelia was one such brave soul.

Stillbirth is the loss of a child after the 20th week of pregnancy. The longer a child is with you, in utero or not, the harder it is to heal from the loss of that child. I have worked with many women over the years who simply cannot wrap their heads around the stillbirths of their children. It can send them into deep states of mental unwellness and depression, and often leaves a wound that is hard to recover from—especially when that stillbirth occurs as your first pregnancy.

Amelia was one of the most complex cases I have ever seen. She explained the tragic story of her loss with the sort of wit that comes from people who have experienced the darkest aspects of life but still managed to live. There is a reason firefighters and first responders are known as jokesters: humor helps dismantle trauma.

Amelia became a midwife after the stillbirth of her child, which occurred in her 20s. Her path of loss and her anger at the insensitivity with which she was treated by the conventional medical system at the time inspired her to help change the story for other women. Years went by, and a subsequent pregnancy resulted in miscarriage. She turned her attention to helping others have healthy pregnancies instead of continuing to try for her own.

But at one point, she changed her mind. "I'm going to be 35 soon," she said. "I've got to try again now, if I am going to ever try again." I was immediately on Amelia's team. I remember both the joy and fear she felt when she discovered she was pregnant. We saw each other almost every week to work through the anxiety and fear of the unknown while also strengthening and supporting her body. Amelia had lost her best friend at a young age, and her young mind and heart had dealt with the loss by becoming obsessive about certain thoughts and behaviors. The loss of her first child was a similar repetition of the grief and complexity she had felt as a child.

When I see repetitive patterns, I look deeper into what these events mean in the greater unfolding story of a person's life. I had the sense that the child that Amelia lost was related to the best friend who'd tragically passed away. By the time she came to see me, it felt like the karmic pattern she had been living in had begun to shift—and part of that was due to the spectacularly strong and present energy of her daughter's spirit.

"This is going to be a successful pregnancy. She is strong and wants to be here," I told Amelia every week. But there were a few times when it felt like the energy of the past tried to creep in, and that the pregnancy was in danger. "I feel like we all barely made it," Amelia told me after the healthy birth of her daughter. The combination of her own faith and love, and the strength of her baby's resolve to be here, persevered and literally dug out a new karmic path for Amelia's life.

## Exercise: *Clearing Unresolved Grief*

Society once had a process and rituals to cushion those who had recently grieved. The tradition of wearing black to alert others that a person was in a period of mourning has been practiced for centuries. Adhering to a ritual mourning period, while also assisting in the smooth transition of a loved one's spirit into the afterlife, is still common in many religious lineages. But what about grief that does not pass or heal with time?

The most important path to avoiding unresolved grief is to allow yourself sufficient time to grieve. Grief has the power to stop a person's unfolding life in its tracks with a chilling slowness; it is not easily shrugged off. This slowness is by design, creating the time and space to process loss. Space and time have become somewhat antithetical to modern life, while grief and melancholy have remained unchanged by technology and digital communication.

Identifying grief is as simple as asking yourself to take an honest inventory of when you have experienced the loss of a friend, a lover, a family member, or even a dream. How much time did you allow yourself to process the grief? Who did you share the loss with, and did you share completely how the loss impacted your life? And, most importantly, how can you allow yourself the time needed to work through and clear unresolved grief now? It is very possible to heal the wounds of the past in the present; in fact, you are better equipped than you were in the past.

The main characters in our lives have this power. They can swoop in and change everything that we thought we knew or understood about ourselves and the universe. They surprise us by being completely different from what we expected or even who we anticipated meeting. Children that are born after particularly difficult periods of spiritual crisis are always gifted healers. They are drawn to wounded people to practice and cultivate their own unique healing powers. In this way, the more honest we are with our children and the less we try to hide and cover up our soul's hurt and pain, the more we set the stage for their learning and practice of compassion. All relationships are karmic relationships.

## EMBRACING THE IMPOSSIBLE

The first and only time I had a past-life regression was at the Berkeley Psychic Institute. I was 26 and already a practicing doctor, but I was still uncertain of my path and its direction and sought out a psychic. I sat before a middle-aged woman who didn't look particularly spiritual; in fact, I remember thinking that she looked like she had just come from a job at a bank or university. The only information I gave her about myself was my name.

After 20 minutes of silent meditation, she spoke. "You have always been a healer," she said. I was shocked. "For many lives, you have practiced medicine. But I see a life in ancient Mongolia. You were a medicine woman and married to a colonel. You were the only woman to travel with the army. They would take you with them to help the injured. But you longed for your child and missed her greatly."

So much of what she said rang true, and I left feeling both awed and reassured. It's not that any of my questions were answered, but the reassurance that a complete stranger could clearly read certain ageless truths about my spirit reminded me that my life was unfolding like it should. I felt that each life I have led was a deepening exploration into the major themes and lessons of my soul, and that there was a divine intelligence working through me.

When I remind people to look at their lives from a larger panoramic perspective, they can often recount the most significant moments in their character and plot development, just like in a movie. Often, we are looking so closely at the goals that are right in front of us that we neglect to relax our gaze to see past the horizon.

Art is one of my favorite metaphors for working with the energetic realm. My daughter made me a beautiful painting in kindergarten. When I asked her to tell me what it was, she shrugged her shoulders and said, "I don't know. It's just an abstract." The true meaning was not in the details but in the kindness and love she felt in wanting to make something just for me.

When you examine grand theories of karma and spiritual contracts, you need to remove the everyday glasses that you see the world through. Sometimes, squinting your eyes just a little and allowing your imagination to fill in the blanks will unveil the magical message hidden within the patterns of your life. You have everything you need to determine the most essential energetics that have been at work in this lifetime and others. Your children, your partner, and your friends and family are an essential part of your karmic circle. As you determine the hidden yet consistent messages from your spirit, it becomes easier to see the similarities in other energetic characters of your life.

## Spiritual Fertility Essentials

Understanding karma is a window into the deepest and most important relationships in our lives, including those with our future children. In this chapter, you learned how the main characters in your life have the power to swoop in and change everything, and that children born after long periods of loss are often gifted healers, a result of the wisdom that comes from suffering. *Karma* literally means action, so when we examine the actions of our lives, we are also examining our karma.

Remember to be observant of these actions and to the timing and unfolding of events in your life. It is only when we gain perspective on the most intense events of our lives that we begin to understand why they happened. The wisdom that comes from surviving loss and grief is often the most valuable wisdom we can gain. But it's not easy to alchemize this material from negative to positive. It takes time and a practice of faith, hope, and love.

# Chapter 10

# The Power of Prayer

Most of the preceding chapters have focused on techniques to identify and remove the filters that disconnect you from your intuition as a path for healing. Prayer is different. While it can connect you to your intuitive wisdom, that is not its ultimate goal or strength.

Prayer is a call for help and an offering of gratitude. Like many of us, I remember to pray when I am scared, and I forget to pray when I am grateful. But it seems only fair to offer up devotion in times of happiness and peace if you use invocation in times of pain and suffering.

I believe that we are all connected, and I also believe that God exists in all life and all consciousness. Because I *know* this, I have seen the power of prayer as it answers a request for help, and I have seen the beauty of prayer as it rises up to rejoice in gratitude. Fertility and the creation of life often call on both types of prayer for support and expression.

Prayer is an art in and of itself, and yet the simplest prayer said with intention and honesty can be as powerful as the well-articulated address or speech. A silent prayer can sometimes be the most powerful of all prayers. A song can be a prayer, and so can a poem or a dance. Some are written, passed down through the millennia, and taught to us as children, in temples, churches, and synagogues. Others exist only for a moment before they are carried away in the wind, seeking the audience they requested.

The gradual loss of a recurring day of rest in Judeo-Christianity, known as the Sabbath (which was used for worship, congregation, and prayer), reveals how full and difficult modern life has become—and how challenging it is to incorporate rest and prayer into our lives. While I understand the necessity of prayer today, I often felt embarrassed as a child when my family would pray in public before meals at restaurants. Being identified in the crowd for my spiritual beliefs and practices was scary. My intuitive nature easily picked up on the judgment of those around us who laughed and rolled their eyes. I tried to leave for the restroom or act like I was not paying attention during the prayer, but there was never any condition in which a mealtime prayer could be missed or skipped. Now more than ever, I understand why ritualistic and habitual prayer is important, especially when it comes to saying grace. I am now just fine sticking out in the crowd, especially for my beliefs and spiritual practices. What I didn't understand as a child was that it never mattered what others thought. Internalizing their commentary was a reflection of my own internal battle between faith and doubt.

Over the years, I have learned to pray in ways that felt meaningful and specific to me. If you grew up praying, you possess a template for how to pray, but you don't have to follow it. Prayer evolves with people's needs and desires, and you are free to express your invocation to the universe however you want.

It's not easy to ask for help, and even more challenging to admit that you might not know what to do next. Prayer is a powerful practice of asking for support, and yet we can be critical of our vulnerability. Self-judgment about prayer is usually residual material from broken-down old beliefs. This also applies to those who did not grow up in a religious or spiritual tradition and never learned how to pray. Just as we forget to ask for help and support from our friends and family, our guides, and our ancestors, we also forget to ask for help from God. We can form attachments to our anxiety and fear. They become friends in chaotic and confusing times, when we grasp on to anything and anyone who can help us feel secure.

Miracles are possible with only one condition: They must be requested. This request is what separates a miracle from all the other tools that you have learned in this book. A miracle is an answer to a prayer, and although God is acting in all moments of life, to catch God's gaze and attention, we simply need ask. Prayer is the ultimate free-fall exercise of trust—the ultimate offering of what is difficult to say in words alone. Ultimately, prayer is what connects us directly to the universe, and it is also how the universe speaks through us.

> ### Exercise: *Request a Miracle*
>
> What can you leave as a sacrifice at the altar? While there are many traditions of lighting candles or placing incense and fruit as offerings on religious altars, this exercise asks you to leave your anxiety, worry, and grief.
>
> Identify the emotions that are weighing you down and blocking your connection to faith and hope. Write each of these worries and concerns on separate pieces of paper. Perhaps you find yourself unable to release anger, jealousy, or envy. One of the most important mantras in healing is to practice not taking things personally. When you do this, you find effective ways to clear attachment to these negative energies.
>
> As you rekindle your personal relationship to the universe through prayer, ask to be given perspective and insight into specific steps to release this energy. When you are ready to give up the worries and concerns that you have written down, find a sacred space to either burn or bury the paper. As you do so, make a trade with the Divine. Request a miracle in exchange for your offering.

## BEYOND THE RATIONAL MIND

In Chapter 3, you read Lacey's story of how she conceived after the trauma of failed IVF by creating a lullaby and connecting to her child's spirit. The creation and practice of song has long been used to unify and connect individuals and groups to the Divine. Some traditions on Earth use song to help bring in the spirit of a child. In certain African tribes, a mother cultivates a lullaby once she feels the call to have a child. She often goes on a vision quest to listen to nature, the spirits of her ancestors, and signs from the heavens. Once she has learned the song of her child, she brings it back to her home and shares it. The song is a prayer of her own hopes to become a mother, but it is also a transmission of her child's energy. I've said before that all mothers are naturally intuitive, but what I really mean is that all mothers are transmitters of universal wisdom.

It's not easy to describe the desire and longing to have a child. It can be all-consuming. Some of this intensity might be a biological imperative, but most of it, from what I have learned, is an extension of human beings' need for love and the desire to share this love. Once upon a time on Earth, according to most spiritual traditions, there existed a state of balance and peace. In many traditional creation myths, humans were made in the reflection of God, and given a plentitude of food and shelter. It was only after becoming more curious about the state of existence that things became difficult for us. The choice to want to know more, while not necessarily good for us, is a hallmark of being human. When I work with new patients, they are often heavily prepared with facts, data, cutting-edge research, and blood panels. They are well aware of the intellectual process of getting pregnant and typically unaware of the internal and unseen process that allows pregnancy to happen. But the desire to share love is present, and this element of the fertility treatment is not ruled by the rational mind. It's ruled by the heart.

We know how to talk to and through the rational mind, but how do you speak to and through the heart? I often use the analogy of writing a poem to describe this. When you sit down to write a poem, you must first connect to the feeling that you are seeking to capture in words. There is a liberty in this that allows you to move beyond the typical rules of language; the grammar and structure of the sentence can be abstract, the words can rhyme (or not), and the length is negotiable. Poetry lives by different rules because poetry is descriptive of something beyond rational thought. Prayer and song, which derive from the heart, are similar.

## PRAYER AS SONG AND POETRY

I describe the act of connecting to the spirit of your child as calling your baby home. When I shared this with my community, my friend Donna Lewis—a successful singer and songwriter by trade—told me that she had a story and a song for me. I soon found myself in Donna's recording studio, where she played me a song she had recorded several years earlier, "Calling In (Fill Up My Mojo)." Then she began to recount how the song came to life.

"I had a miscarriage," she confessed. "I was living back in the U.K., and it was a particularly difficult and scary event." She went on to describe her subsequent grief, sadness, and struggle to heal from the loss. "A healer over there helped me see that I needed to allow the spirit of that child to leave. We went to the ocean and had a ritual to let go." Soon after, Donna moved to the U.S. full-time and began to consider getting pregnant again. She was well into her 40s at this time, and felt discouraged by doctors who just saw her age and not her overall health and being.

"I started really caring for myself. Filled up my mojo," she said. "I found a wonderful Eastern medicine practitioner who believed in my body and ability to conceive and have a healthy pregnancy, and I continued to do the spiritual work, as well. I practiced having faith and hope. I wrote this song during that time as an expression of this faith and hope."

The lyrics to this powerful anthem, just like a prayer, were devotional and filled with longing and desire, as well as joy and courage. As she was writing the song, Donna had scheduled an appointment at the local reproductive fertility clinic—she ended up canceling as she found out she was pregnant. A powerful verse in her song had foreshadowed this pregnancy: "Come on, sing in my dreams, I'm giving up the machines, I know I'm ready, I can really do this." And she did.

Song shares much in common with prayer. Words and mantras can be repeated in rhythm and harmony to elicit a feeling or state of consciousness. The hymns that people sing in church and temple are often prayers set to music. Sound therapy is an ancient practice that opens and heals blocked energy and emotion in the body while excavating the unconscious. The lullaby itself is designed to assist in the transition from conscious and waking life to the unconscious and dreaming world. I love the use of poetry and song to offer up the anxiety, fear, joy, and intensity of the path to parenthood—especially for those who have difficulty digesting their skepticism about a universal consciousness or spiritual practice.

## PRAYER AS A SACRED SPACE

Many years after the West Texas drive that I described in the beginning of this book, and soon after trying to conceive, I felt the spirit of my daughter enter my body while sitting in one of the most sacred places on Earth. There are a few places, most of which are in nature, that I refer to as my spiritual homes. We all have them, but sometimes we forget to name and recognize their power. They are spaces where we feel most connected to our spirit, to our guides, and to God. It's easy to pray here because every word and every step feels sacred. Sacré-Coeur is one such place for me.

The cathedral of Sacré-Coeur was built in the late 19th century and is perched atop a long-occupied hill overlooking Paris. It is a place where I travel when I am in need of guidance. Painted on the roof of the cathedral is a large mural dedicated to the sacred heart of Jesus, as well as the saints that protect France, including Mary and Joan of Arc. At the time, this interpretation of Christ was influenced by a new idea of Jesus as a compassionate and all-forgiving force. But this landmark to Christianity was built on a site that had a long history in France. Before becoming a home to bohemians and artists, the French Resistance of World War II was headquartered in the surrounding neighborhood; and long before that, it had been occupied by the Romans. For me, the metaphor of the sacred perched in the center of rebellion and art resonates deeply. And the conscious orchestration of environment and timing contributed to setting the stage to welcome my daughter to the planet.

The sacred space of the body can be prepared for pregnancy through the physical and the spiritual realms. Spending time in sacred spaces, such as temples, churches, forests, or beaches, encourages the body to mirror the energy by which it is surrounded. Spaces that encourage prayer are sacred spaces. One's birthplace influences many factors of a person's constitution, as do season and year.

As an example, I was born at West Point Military Academy. My father was finishing his career in the military, and it was one of the last places he was stationed. Although I only lived there the first years of my life, my earliest memories are of walking along stone fences against the backdrop

of the Hudson River. West Point is a place that has histor-
ically trained warriors and military leaders in American
history. The place resonates with who I am, with certain
qualities of my spirit, as the past-life therapist described
in a previous chapter. Ironically, decades later, after a
move from central Texas to New York City, I find myself
living very close, as the crow flies, to my West Point. Like
a migratory animal, I made my way back home. As I have
witnessed my daughter's personality and spirit bloom, I
see the rich tapestry of Sacré-Coeur and Montmartre in
her character. She is rebellious, artistic, and expressive
while being simultaneously kind and openhearted.

Likewise, in Hawaii there is a tradition of women traveling to specific sites in nature, watched over by ancestor
spirits and gods, to give birth. These Hawaiian birth sites
are located in several power spots on each island, and they
archived generation upon generation of past births before
the current hospital model took hold.

My dear friend Lucia Horan, an energetic alchemist
and spiritual teacher, gave birth on Maui. "I had to fight
fiercely for a natural birth," she recollected. The birth of
her daughter was empowered by Lucia's lineage of connection and trust in the body and the spirit. "What's crazy,"
Lucia noted, "is that Hawaii has one of the highest C-
section rates in the U.S." How could a culture with such
a rich history of birth rites and practices trade it all so
quickly for a medicalized birth in a sterile environment?
"It reflects the injury to the people's spirit that happened
through colonization," she continued. "But there is a
movement to change this. Sadly, one of the local birthing
sites, which was in a luscious valley, was literally turned
into a dump. But people are beginning to clean it up and
repair it."

The metaphor is crystal clear. Trauma impacts our physical environment, as well as our mental and psychological environment. But nothing of the spirit can ever truly be lost, just buried and hidden. It waits to be activated and rekindled when the time is right.

## Exercise: *Find Your Spiritual Home*

We often stack the odds against ourselves, creating reasons why something cannot occur instead of focusing on our powers to manifest and create. We can change this by beginning to look around at our environment, home, and city. Do you live in or frequently visit a place that helps your spirit thrive, or is your environment a reflection of a sadness and melancholy that you embody?

Find a space that you consider holy and sacred, and spend as much time there as possible. If you have been drawn to a sacred space that is in another town, state, or country but are unsure how to get there, I recommend having a conversation with your future self. Envision residing in the place you seek to live. Ask your future self very specific questions as to what you need to do right now to get there, and start to implement these steps. This is also a powerful tool for visualizing your future children and the timeline of their arrival.

### PRAYER AS A SACRED TOOL FOR NAMING

The components of consciously entering into parenthood are unique to each individual and couple. Preparation of the body, mind, and spirit looks different for everyone. Paying attention to time, place, season, and environment is a really good start. The process of choosing a name for your baby is also an act of setting sacred space and sending your prayers out to the universe.

When we choose a name for a child, we can look at the past and the ancestors who came before us. We can look at the influence of the season and month, such as summer or the month of April. And we can acknowledge the place, such as Paris, a spot next to a river, a mountain, or the ocean.

The act of choosing a child's name is an expression of consciousness. A name has to *feel* right for a person. Just like poetry and prayer, the word has to capture the descriptive feeling that is that person and be an offering between Earth and heaven. To capture the spirit of my daughter, my husband and I chose the name Anna Libertine. Anna means "of God," and Libertine, "free of morality and law." She is certainly both.

Acknowledging with words is a form of naming. The use of language to express that which is sacred can be seen in the practice of naming an individual or in describing the places on Earth where we feel most in alignment, at peace and unified with spirit. Some people's names are received by their parents or a family member through the nonrational mind, sometimes in a dream or a vision. Prayer is similar to both of these practices. Prayer can be simple or complex. It can be a call for help or a deep request when in need. Any time we pray, we enter into a sacred space of connection—not only with the universe but with our own spirits, as well.

## IT'S OKAY TO NOT KNOW

Rose had suffered through a long road of unsuccessful fertility treatments. After many rounds of IVF and miscarriage, her medical team made the decision to start looking at the option of a donor egg. Premature ovarian failure can happen at any time, but for Rose, its early onset by age 29 was particularly saddening.

Rose, although complex, is my favorite type of client to assist. Within her story were layers of trauma from the emotional, physical, and spiritual planes. And while she could identify each of these traumas, no one in particular stood out as the root cause of her infertility.

Intense and unexplainable phenomena that occur to us in life can be soul-crushing. In many spiritual traditions, there is an outlet to understand this "randomness" by placing faith in God. While the suffering will continue, the mind can, at the minimum, stop incessantly trying to understand why such events occurred if it accepts this faith in God's ultimate plan.

Rose was unsure about how to proceed. "I just don't know what God wants for me," she said. While a donor egg was a potential path (and, Rose reasoned, "at least it would be my husband's child"), she was unsure if she was ready to take that step. Rose had grown up in a home in which her father repeatedly cheated on her mother, and each time her mother took him back and forgave him, it was at the expense of her own self-esteem. "My father even had a secret child that I didn't find out about until I was 17," she shared. In Rose's mind, having her own family was supposed to help her heal from the trauma of her own childhood. She was afraid that if she carried another woman's egg, anger and jealousy would ruin the pregnancy and her relationship. Rose worried using someone else's genetic material would make her feel inferior, and questioned if she was repeating patterns of the past instead of healing that hurt.

The choice to use a donor egg or sperm is not necessarily an easy one. Many of my clients have had difficulty with the decision and come to me for intuitive counsel. They are almost always surprised when they hear that I am supportive of the use of another person's genetic material, with certain stipulations. The more involved science is in the conception, the more you need to counterbalance the rational with the spiritual. The story of your child's conception and the preparation around it must be led by the practice of consciousness and a practice of spirit. After all, any place can serve as a space to practice the sacred, as long as the conditions are correct. The most sacred text can be carried in a brown paper bag, a backpack, or a fine leather suitcase. It's how you handle the material inside that matters most.

I asked Rose to pray, specifically for guidance on the events of her life and for clarity on how to proceed. I often say that the first God you know is always the God you know best. I knew she had grown up Catholic, and although she was no longer practicing, she still walked along a strong path of faith.

After several months, Rose returned with God's response: "We are adopting!"

"You are?" I responded with enthusiasm.

She explained, "After I left our last session, I went across the street to the church to pray. I lit a candle and asked God for guidance and promised to listen to what I heard with faith. On the way out, I saw a flyer about volunteer work in Guatemala, and I took a picture and looked up more details when I got home. Honestly, I was so lost,

I wanted a break from my own life and drama. So I signed up to volunteer."

Rose's husband supported the idea, and they decided they would meet in Costa Rica after her week volunteering. "We never made it to Costa Rica," she said. "I hadn't realized that I had signed up to work in an orphanage. We were just meant to help the local diocese with whatever they needed and God sent me to an orphanage—and more importantly, God sent me to my daughter."

Although Rose had never considered adoption, when she held an orphaned newborn baby girl in the orphanage, she immediately connected and recognized the baby's story as her own. She called her husband that day and told him to get on the next flight to Guatemala. She told me, "I might still pursue fertility treatments later, but for now, I have found the child God intended us to have. I have no doubt in my heart that everything in my life led up to the moment I walked into that orphanage and met her."

## GOD KNOWS

Until the mid-1960s, when you asked a woman how many children she wanted to have, her answer would most likely be, "God knows." Ask the same question now, and most people will have very specific numbers, with sex and timing planned far in advance. While all of this can be helpful, as soon as these desires cross into the material world, they can become mere objectives to achieve with a great deal of effort as opposed to possible outcomes we can shepherd in with ease.

Many of my patients, while very spiritual, express feeling alienated by the religious systems they have left behind. It can sometimes be hard for them to rekindle a faith-based practice. In my own life, although my parents are very supportive of my choices and philosophy, there remains a judgment about the way my actions have broken with their religious beliefs. I have felt the pain of not being able to share with my parents my spiritual studies or the miraculous systems of intuitive medicine that I have learned and practiced. It has been difficult for me to understand how people who have such faith and belief in God are incapable or even afraid of systems of healing that deviate from the Western allopathic model. But as my mother recently said, "When we were growing up, the mind was split from the body, and both were split from the spirit."

To me, compartmentalizing these three aspects of consciousness simply doesn't work. And so I responded, "How do you show your faith in God when the first place you run when suffering is not the church but the doctor's office?" That said, I do believe organized religion has been a very powerful tool for teaching the world how to recognize and participate in the sacred. Without it, while we are free to choose and create independently, we run the risk of forgetting to pray.

Part of emotional maturity is learning how to bracket the strong beliefs of others and to see how those beliefs are a part of their projections, and not yours. In fact, I think learning not to take things personally is essential for spiritual liberation, a jewel of wisdom that I learned in the first few years of my daughter's life. And yet, no matter what, certain relatives and close friends will always have the ability to trigger shame and guilt, especially if they can back up these judgments with religious or social law.

Is there a way to return to a deeper trust in the universe, without blindly and unquestioningly accepting religious mandates?

There are opportunities in each of our life paths, especially in the fertility process, to examine our lives, our actions, and our spirit. The window into self-knowledge and reconnection to faith, hope, and love is essential. During the vulnerable times of our life, when our armor is weakened, when we are forlorn, sick, and in despair, we are often the most honest. The access this honesty provides is a chance to pray and offer up the weight that is too much for one person to carry.

I believe that we will, together, "get back to the garden." Our children will remember the path there, not by looking at maps and GPS coordinates, but by living a life that reflects the principles of the garden: namely, love for others, compassion, care for the Earth, and appreciation for art and beauty. Their ability to actualize this is directly related to the work you do in your lifetime, both before they are born and after. The tone you set, the song and prayer that resonates through your life, is a part of the harmonization of all life on Earth.

## Spiritual Fertility Essentials

This chapter described the processes of prayer, which is one of the most powerful fertility tools available to you. It reflects the interconnectedness that unifies all of us here on Earth and the heavens. Prayer can deliver magic into your life, but you must ask for help to receive it. This may seem like an obvious practice; however, it is one of the hardest to implement consistently in our lives. When you incorporate prayer into your life, either through routine or ritual, you gain access to a sacred space where you are able to shed some of the weight that you are carrying with you. Most of the time, this excess stress is a byproduct from your rational mind and overthinking, but prayer can powerfully remove this from your heart and mind. Prayer likewise prepares the sacred space of your body for pregnancy. Spending time in cathedrals, temples, and the church of nature will facilitate the practice of prayer, however you wish to engage in it.

# Conclusion

# The Future of Fertility

All journeys of healing begin with self-examination. In this process, we usually ask a similar set of questions as to why, how, and what occurred in the past that led us into a current state of being unwell. The symptom, after all, is a branch of our complete being; what is most essential is the entire tree and the health of the root.

When we talk about fertility, we are speaking about more than an individual's journey. An individual is like a branch that is connected to other branches and grounded through the trunk and the roots of our collective consciousness on Earth. Each symptom opens a window for introspection and healing. As we individually do the *work* of healing, we simultaneously heal past and future generations, wounds in our cultures, and our relationship to the numinous. I've worked as a healer for two decades, and what I have found in that time is that the most powerful example of this window into healing occurs within fertility.

Human beings are stewards of the Earth. Many traditions on the planet also say that we were made in the image of God and that our responsibility is greater than that of other living beings because of this likeness. For so many of us, consciousness is a heavy crown. It is easy to look back at failed attempts made by groups of the past who tried to create new ways of living in harmony with the Earth. Many of the collective living models championed in the 1960s and 1970s that incorporated compassion, environmentalism, and collective creation failed miserably when put to the test. Religious communities often sacrifice the happiness and expression of the individual to create a more unified and harmonized group. Politics is in a perpetual duel. The left battles the right and the right battles the left, when all the while it's the people in the middle who suffer and are lost.

But this doesn't have to be the case. We continue to learn from our mistakes. We must pass through failed models of religion, politics, and economics in order to truly learn what works and what doesn't. Although it might not be obvious, things on Earth are getting better— but that doesn't mean that any of us can sit back and rest. If anything, we have to work harder than ever.

## HELPING THE GOOD INTO THE WORLD

A few years ago, I went on a spiritual pilgrimage to the rain forest of Costa Rica. It was the longest amount of time I had been away from my daughter, and it was emotionally very difficult. I was anxious and fearful that she would be vulnerable without my presence and that something bad might happen to her without me close by. I realized that time away from the people I'm most attached to was essential for my growth. I was reminded of the primary relationship that we explored in Chapter 4: the one between me and the universe. I remembered that the people whom we are tied to through love and spirit are always with us, even through distance, death, and time. I could love my daughter and my husband more honestly, more deeply, when I let go of my attachments and viewed them without the filters of conditionality.

Sitting next to the fire under the moon in one of the last great biodiverse places on Earth, the healer I had traveled to study under asked me why I did the work of fertility. "I care about women having healthy pregnancies and healthy children," I responded.

"Yes, but what's beyond that?" she asked.

"I care about consciousness and healing," I said.

Still one more time, she asked, "Why do you do the work you do?"

Several sets of eyes were on me as my own began to tear. I exhaled and said, "I have to keep helping the good come into the world, because there is so much bad just waiting to take over. When a child is born through consciousness and love, they help tip the scales to the light."

As much as I am meant to be a mother and a partner in this lifetime, these relationships are only extensions of my soul's purpose and path. I identify as my daughter's mother, but this identity is representative of something timeless between her soul and mine. I have faith that the soul work that she and I accomplish independently in this lifetime is more important than our personal relationship. Before she was born, I thought that the shift into being a mother would somehow change me. And it did, but not in the way that I thought. Becoming a parent is never what you think it will be. If anything, it is an opportunity to be spiritually initiated, to pass through the systems that worked in the past but have since become irrelevant. The tighter you hold on to the old ways, the old you, the longer the transformation takes. Like the Earth, we are constantly evolving, and the only thing certain is change.

I see each of us as spiritual beings. And I see each of us as powerful manifestors who have traded in these abilities for the comfort of knowing. And while it is true that knowing is a great tool for defending and planning for the future, the future still comes regardless of what you comprehend and how well you comprehend it. Strengthening the spirit is the best practice for preparing for the future. A spirit that is nurtured when life is balanced and calm is ready for the times of chaos and turbulence.

I offer this statement to the reader who has suffered through the long and toilsome fertility journey. The depth of self-knowledge that is gained in the waiting, in the fertility treatments themselves, in the self-doubt and despair, powerfully strengthens your spirit, eternally. The greatest danger that threatens this hard-earned wisdom comes in the form of loss of faith, love, and hope. While I have offered several tools in this book to help protect your spirit, ultimately it is your own courage that matters most. Digging deep to abolish the despair along your path requires you to keep dreaming and keep believing that better days will come. This might sometimes seem impossible, but look around. We all share the vision on Earth that someday it, too, will be better. If we didn't believe this, even unconsciously, none of us would continue to work as hard as we do or love as deeply.

When individuals radically heal their life, everyone around them is impacted. The same is inversely true when someone takes his or her own life. The dynamic power of healing radiates outward and reveals a path that others who might not think themselves capable of healing can follow. I have seen entire families healed by the birth of one child, but the path of spiritual fertility is about far more than conceiving or the choice to become a parent. The life that we live is a model for others, including friends and family, our children and future children, and our grandchildren.

## RECOGNIZING THE POWER OF COLLECTIVE CONSCIOUSNESS

I've spoken throughout this book about collective consciousness. As much as I am an advocate of the individual, I think our untapped power on Earth will be accessed when each and every one of us has the opportunity and experience of individuation. Individuality is the cornerstone of modern economics, marketing, and media—and although we have platforms to express ourselves to the world regardless of location, age, or nationality, many on the planet are still limited by poverty, sexual expression, and war. People, especially those of us who have been privileged to be free, are beginning to recognize that individual freedom can only take us so far. Without a greater connection to our community, and in an environment where many of us are not granted the same opportunities, our growth remains atrophied. When we stress individuality over community, we remain isolated and unaware of our full capacity to love and be loved.

"I want my greatest achievement to be the children I have raised," said my dear friend and accomplished colleague, Dr. Jennifer Ashby, with whom I met at an international fertility conference as I was writing this section of the book.

"Yes," I responded, "but you raise your children to be individuals of service. You raise them to be aware of the collective consciousness of Earth."

"I do, but what's the alternative?" Jennifer asked.

"I think most people raise children to be an extension of themselves," I replied. "They expect their kids to pick up where they left off or finish the achievements they never did."

What if we began conceiving and raising children not only for ourselves but for humanity? What would it look like if we supported one another through pregnancy and the raising of children because we recognized the power of the collective instead of only the power and desire of the individual?

If you recall Kate's story in Chapter 5, her struggle with the choice to have a child or save the planet almost kept her from becoming a mother—but she discovered that it did not have to be that way. Kate found that her passion and mission to protect the Earth was intertwined with a deep respect for motherhood itself. When we bring consciousness and spiritual practice into conception and parenthood, we build the infrastructure for human beings to be sovereign and unique, while also understanding that they are not alone and that they are an integral part of something far greater. I have learned this by watching the children whom I have helped bring to Earth, as they grow and thrive. They are each beautiful and radiant in their energy. The love and consciousness from which they were born has engendered in them something dynamic and powerful. However, it shouldn't be that only some children have access to this support. Everyone, especially those who are the most disadvantaged on the planet as well as the ones who cannot ask for advocacy, should not be expected to give voice to their suffering. When a person is a victim of their family and their culture, we have a duty to step in and offer help, even if it is not requested.

Years ago, as I mentioned in an earlier chapter, I did a residency on a labor and delivery floor at a busy hospital in Shanghai. I arrived late Sunday night on a direct flight from New York City and barely slept before my first morning at the hospital. I was with a small group of doctors, and our translator, who was supposed to meet us at the hospital, was late. Hospitals are publicly run in China, and the high population means that they are also very crowded.

I put on scrubs, washed my hands, and walked into a large triage room with 16 laboring women all in different stages of labor. We joined the doctor on call for rounds as, in broken English, he quickly explained each patient's condition. In the back right corner, a beautiful young woman was breathing heavily yet rhythmically, with her eyes closed.

"She's almost in transition," the doctor said.

As we continued, I noticed a patient who was crying and visibly upset. She appeared to be six months pregnant. Concerned for her health, I asked the doctor about her condition.

"This is a chemical abortion," he replied coldly and moved on.

Confused and overwhelmed, we were ushered into a long hallway, where we sat. Not much time passed before both of the women I mentioned were simultaneously wheeled out of the triage room and into the main delivery room down the hall. In China and many places in the world, the concept of a private delivery suite is unheard of. This room was very warm and had enough space for several laboring women at a time. It was staffed by nurses, a midwife, and a medical doctor. Between the jet lag and the culture shock, everything felt unreal that morning. And as I observed a perfectly healthy and beautiful baby boy born to the stoic and brave young woman, I concurrently observed, just four or five feet away, the medically induced stillbirth of a baby girl. Neither woman seemed to acknowledge the other, and it was all business as usual to the medical staff. But for me, the juxtaposition of these two births was deeply moving.

Later, the translator arrived and I asked him to find out why the termination had taken place, expecting a medical reason to be the cause. "Family politics," he told me with a sigh. "She did not want the abortion."

For many people on the planet, the choice of reproductive freedom is not much of a choice at all. "Family politics" for the woman in despair was code for the fact that a girl child was not wanted by her family, and that without the support of her family, she had no option for raising a child on her own. She had no choice, nor any spiritual or psychological support.

## HEALING THROUGH COMPASSION, NONJUDGMENT, AND SERVICE TO OTHERS

I share this story because it is one of the events of my life that has most impacted the way I practice fertility medicine. And while it describes a story that many would consider sad, I share it because things are actually getting better on this planet. The repression of women that long went unspoken within society has now been brought to light, and the transgressors who were once safe in the shadows are no longer able to remain unknown. While I work tirelessly to help each of my patients heal trauma and blockages, and to connect with the spirits of their children, I also do my best to remind each of them that our individual actions and beliefs impact the collective. I teach that exercising an ethic of compassion, nonjudgment, and service to others—especially those who are suffering—is an essential step in healing their own individual fertility.

We are far more connected than we acknowledge. What happens on the other side of the world, regardless if we are aware or not, impacts us. The "heaven" of cheap goods and clothing at your local mall is the "hell" of a child laborer in Asia. The hell of a forced termination and the impact on a woman's soul is felt everywhere, especially by the most empathetic among us.

We have to start caring about more than ourselves, our immediate family, and our own children. The path of spiritual fertility will help you to conceive and will connect you to your child's spirit, but it will also lead you to another type of conception of consciousness, one that I encourage you to share with the world. What you discover about your unique relationship to the universe is a piece of the grand puzzle—and a very important one, at that. Nourish it and continue to practice the steps of this book, long after your child is born.

This book is my transmission to you. It is the piece of the puzzle that I found as I made my way back to belief while helping children to be born in health, spirit, and consciousness. I have faith in your intuitive wisdom, and I am eternally, as I often tell my patients, on your side.

# Acknowledgments

At the age of 14, I wanted to be a writer. My uncle, a professional author, heard this and pulled me into his study to say, "Take any book off the shelf, sit down, and type it. If you can do that, then you can be a writer." He was correct. The discipline and patience it takes to write does not come easily. But the capacity to write is only half of the story of a book. Without the support of people who can see an author's vision, even when it is half conceived, a book remains displaced, like a meteorite searching for a planet and a home. *Spiritual Fertility* found its home at Hay House, and in hindsight, I can say that there was never another path for it. The lineage of authors who have walked the path that Louise Hay paved is one that I feel extremely honored to be a part of.

During my first meeting at Hay House, I sat across the table from my dream team, one of whose members was auspiciously pregnant. As I laid out the concept and theory behind the book, instead of the skepticism I had experienced from other publishing houses, I was welcomed with enthusiasm and brilliant questions. I knew about five minutes into the meeting that Patty Gift, Sally Mason-Swaab, and Richelle Fredson were women that I needed on this book's side. Sally, thank you for your steady energy, compassionate heart, and insightful comments and support along the way. Richelle, thank you for seeing the need and importance of this book and being its advocate. And to Mary Norris, a heartfelt thank you for adding your years of experience to *Spiritual Fertility*. It is a better book because of you. The ethic of professional yet innovative and courageous spirit that I felt from the very first e-mail with Patty Gift is what makes Hay House different from the others. Thank you for continuing to search out and support the much-needed alternative perspectives in healing and spirituality.

Visualization is a powerful tool within manifestation. And while I knew that this book would be written, I needed help finding the path from the here and now to the future. I asked for an intuitive guide and found one in Nirmala Nataraj. Nirmala, you are truly a book doula and one of the smartest people I know. Thank you for being a time traveler with me.

I started the search for representation of this book the morning that I dropped my daughter off for her first day of kindergarten. I didn't know what to expect from the half dozen or so e-mails that I sent out to literary agents around the United States, of which all were women—except for one man. I said a prayer, asking that the person who was meant to help the book would read the book proposal and deeply understand the work. I had been told that it could take weeks to receive feedback, so I was shocked when 20 minutes later I answered a call from Steven Harris, who said with enthusiasm that this book needed to be written and that he would love to be a part of that process. There isn't any better feedback for a first-time author than the support and belief of a fantastic literary agent. Thank you for seeing the vision, Steven.

In listing the many people for whom I am grateful, I can't leave out the energetic support I have received from my ancestors. Their watchful gaze has ushered me gently through the devastating times in my life and led me through open doors and safe passages. To my father, who taught me the importance of keeping a journal, and my mother, who transcribed word after word of my father's writing—thank you for setting an example of a spiritual life of service that could be captured in words. To my family and friends, many of whom are mentioned in the stories of this book, your encouragement and kindness fuel me to keep going and remind me that even if the world sometimes doesn't understand me, you do—and that is all that ultimately matters. There is a special place in my heart for those who provided the support system for our daughter over the first years of her life. To all the teachers, grandparents, caretakers, and friends who step in to support children, you are instrumental in helping women like me to actualize the dream of being a mother while still pursuing our other life's work.

To my patients, the people that I have had the honor to work with, seeing you heal and meet your children is my daily reminder of joy. Thank you for allowing me to share your stories with the world. I'm forever in awe of the depths of the human spirit and capacity to love, even after heartbreak. Witnessing this through your lives and your healing is like reading the greatest book ever written. Your character arcs, your integrity, and the way you navigate the shadows and the light continually bring tears to my eyes. I cried through half the writing of this book, just remembering the magic and beauty that is you. Thank you.

Lastly, to the person I most take for granted but without whom this work could simply not exist: my extraordinarily brilliant husband, Dr. Scott Von. The standard you set for yourself through your work as a doctor, thinker, artist, and healer has been my inspiration since the first day we met. Every time I feel discouraged for being different, you teach me how to counter judgment with intellect and reflection. Each time my intuitive spirit is injured by the world, you defend me, while reminding me that I, too, have the power to speak up and back. You are the true advocate for the outsider and the most intuitively intelligent person I have ever known. I have learned much from being your colleague, but I have learned even more from being your wife. Our daughter inspired this work years before we met. But none of this, including the daily pride I have in being her mother, would have occurred without you and that fated I Ching reading years ago. You and Anna are simply my everything.

# About the Author

Dr. Julie Von is a Manhattan-based holistic doctor specializing in fertility. At a young age, she began apprenticing with healers, shamans, and doctors around the world. Julie became one of the youngest people in the United States to study Chinese medicine and continued her education in China, obtaining an esteemed doctoral degree. Her clinical work in New York City has spanned over a decade and has aligned her with some of the most advanced and well-known names in the field of fertility medicine. Julie merges her medical education with her initiation into Earth-based and intuitive-based practices.

The method called spiritual fertility, which she has developed, has assisted countless couples in conceiving and carrying healthy children into the world.

Julie's unique capacity and experience within both reproductive medicine and medical intuition makes her an extraordinary advocate for her clients. The energetic and intuitive work she shares is grounded in real clinical and medical experience. Julie's work has been called evocative, eloquent, mystical, and practical. Her most sincere desire is to help individuals to connect to the spirits of their children while guiding them to Earth in the most gentle and loving of ways. She lives with her husband and daughter in New York City, the Hudson River Valley, and Malibu. Learn more at drjulievon.com.

We hope you enjoyed this Hay House book. If you'd like to receive our online catalog featuring additional information on Hay House books and products, or if you'd like to find out more about the Hay Foundation, please contact:

Hay House, Inc., P.O. Box 5100, Carlsbad, CA 92018-5100
(760) 431-7695 or (800) 654-5126
(760) 431-6948 (fax) or (800) 650-5115 (fax)
www.hayhouse.com® • www.hayfoundation.org

———

**Published in Australia by:**
Hay House Australia Pty. Ltd., 18/36 Ralph St., Alexandria NSW 2015
*Phone:* 612-9669-4299 • *Fax:* 612-9669-4144 • www.hayhouse.com.au

**Published in the United Kingdom by:**
Hay House UK, Ltd., Astley House, 33 Notting Hill Gate, London W11 3JQ
*Phone:* 44-20-3675-2450 • *Fax:* 44-20-3675-2451 • www.hayhouse.co.uk

**Published in India by:** Hay House Publishers India,
Muskaan Complex, Plot No. 3, B-2, Vasant Kunj, New Delhi 110 070
*Phone:* 91-11-4176-1620 • *Fax:* 91-11-4176-1630 • www.hayhouse.co.in

———

### Access New Knowledge.
### Anytime. Anywhere.

Learn and evolve at your own pace
with the world's leading experts.

www.hayhouseU.com

# Free e-newsletters
# from Hay House, the Ultimate
# Resource for Inspiration

**Be the first to know about Hay House's free downloads, special offers, giveaways, contests, and more!**

 Get exclusive excerpts from our latest releases and videos from *Hay House Present Moments*.

 Our *Digital Products Newsletter* is the perfect way to stay up-to-date on our latest discounted eBooks, featured mobile apps, and Live Online and On Demand events.

 Learn with real benefits! *HayHouseU.com* is your source for the most innovative online courses from the world's leading personal growth experts. Be the first to know about new online courses and to receive exclusive discounts.

 Enjoy uplifting personal stories, how-to articles, and healing advice, along with videos and empowering quotes, within *Heal Your Life*.

## Sign Up Now!

*Get inspired, educate yourself, get a complimentary gift, and share the wisdom!*

**Visit www.hayhouse.com/newsletters to sign up today!**

# Hay House Podcasts
## *Bring Fresh, Free Inspiration Each Week!*

Hay House proudly offers a selection of life-changing audio content via our most popular podcasts!

### Hay House Meditations Podcast

Features your favorite Hay House authors guiding you through meditations designed to help you relax and rejuvenate. Take their words into your soul and cruise through the week!

### Dr. Wayne W. Dyer Podcast

Discover the timeless wisdom of Dr. Wayne W. Dyer, world-renowned spiritual teacher and affectionately known as "the father of motivation." Each week brings some of the best selections from the 10-year span of Dr. Dyer's talk show on HayHouseRadio.com.

### Hay House World Summit Podcast

Over 1 million people from 217 countries and territories participate in the massive online event known as the Hay House World Summit. This podcast offers weekly mini-lessons from World Summits past as a taste of what you can hear during the annual event, which occurs each May.

### Hay House Radio Podcast

Listen to some of the best moments from HayHouseRadio.com, featuring expert authors such as Dr. Christiane Northrup, Anthony William, Caroline Myss, James Van Praagh, and Doreen Virtue discussing topics such as health, self-healing, motivation, spirituality, positive psychology, and personal development.

### Hay House Live Podcast

Enjoy a selection of insightful and inspiring lectures from Hay House Live, an exciting event series that features Hay House authors and leading experts in the fields of alternative health, nutrition, intuitive medicine, success, and more! Feel the electricity of our authors engaging with a live audience, and get motivated to live your best life possible!

Find Hay House podcasts on iTunes, or visit www.HayHouse.com/podcasts for more info.